the BELLY FAT *Diet*

John Chatham

ROCKRIDGE UNIVERSITY PRESS

For general information on our other products and services or to obtain technical support, please contact our Customer Care Department within the U.S. at (866) 744-2665, or outside the U.S. at (510) 253-0500.

Rockridge University Press publishes its books in a variety of electronic and print formats. Some content that appears in print may not be available in electronic books, and vice versa.

ISBN: 978-1-62315-021-1

CONTENTS

Getting Started with Belly Fat Loss

- Introduction to the Belly Fat Diet

- The Dangers of Excess Belly Fat

- What You Can Expect from the Belly Fat Diet

- Everything We Thought Was Wrong: Blasting the Myths about Belly Fat

(1)

INTRODUCTION TO THE BELLY FAT DIET

A flat abdomen has always been the icon of fitness, good health and attractiveness. Every day, there are new diets, workouts and exercise equipment products geared towards losing belly fat and achieving flat, sexy abs.

But losing belly fat isn't just about looking good; it's about being healthy. We now know that excess belly fat is a huge indicator of overall health, especially the risks of heart disease, diabetes and stroke. Losing stored belly fat not only makes you look great and feel better about yourself, it lowers your risk for several diseases and conditions that can greatly affect and even shorten your life.

For decades, getting flat abs was viewed as something that required a great deal of hard work and deprivation. Even people who were fairly fit and active complained that they just couldn't shed that tummy pooch or extra five pounds around their middles. Most people attack that stubborn area with thousands of crunches and one new diet after another, and then become frustrated when there are no new results.

The great news is that in the last five years, we've had so much new research into how and why our bodies both store and use belly fat. Studies done by respected doctors, nutritionists and scientists have revealed that losing stubborn belly fat isn't necessarily about calories, fat grams or crunches. In fact, they've pretty much thrown out all of the things we used to believe about losing belly fat and getting a flat, toned stomach.

Fortunately, that research has also proven that losing belly fat can actually be much faster, easier and more pleasant than anything we used to believe. It doesn't require starvation, hours in the gym or any fancy gadgets or equipment.

The Belly Fat Diet has distilled all of the new research results into one, easy-to-follow plan to help you finally lose that excess fat around your waistline. Best of all, you can do it without being hungry, without spending hours working out or without spending a ton of money on supplements, gym memberships or equipment. You'll eat as much as you want whenever you're hungry, work out as little as twenty minutes per day and feel energized and satisfied.

By following the Belly Fat Diet plan, you'll get dramatic results faster than you ever thought possible and you'll do it without being miserable or sacrificing your health.

We'll provide you with the science behind losing belly fat, as well as a food and shopping guide, recipes, meal plans and a workout program that you'll customize just for you. All you'll need is a commitment to change your body and your health for the better!

Measure Your Risk: *A waist measurement of more than half your height in inches indicates serious risk of heart disease, stroke and diabetes. To measure your waist properly, use a measuring tape to measure the circumference of your waist at the belly button. A woman who is 5'4" (64 inches) and has a waist measurement of 32 inches or more is at serious risk of developing these health problems.*

2

THE DANGERS OF EXCESS BELLY FAT

During a recent television appearance, renowned cardiologist and author Dr. Mehmet Oz caused quite a stir by announcing that your waist measurement is the most important indicator of overall health. During the show, he explained that if your waist measurement is more than half your height (in inches), you are at serious risk for heart disease, stroke and type 2 diabetes. This announcement had many people looking at their measuring tapes not just as a way to measure their fitness, but as a way to measure their future.

Why is excess belly fat so important and what does it have to do with all of these health risks?

Excess Belly Fat Damages Your Liver

Several recent studies on the connection between obesity (particularly excess belly fat) and high levels of liver fat have shown that there is a much higher rate of fatty liver in those with excess belly fat. Fatty liver is a leading indicator of several lipid and metabolic disorders and even liver cancer. In these studies, researchers investigated what makes some obese people develop lipid disorders. They found that liver fat is strongly associated with increased secretion of very low density lipoproteins (VLDL), which contain the highest amount of triglycerides. High levels of triglycerides carry an increased risk of metabolic abnormalities and increased risk of heart disease and premature death.

Decreasing excess belly fat and blood cholesterol is the recommended treatment for reducing and even reversing fatty liver.

Excess Belly Fat Increases Insulin Resistance and Type 2 diabetes

When we eat, our food, especially carbohydrates, is broken down into glucose so that it can be used to power every cell in our bodies. However, to be used as energy rather than stored as fat, glucose requires the help of insulin.

Insulin is a hormone secreted by the pancreas. Its job is to serve as a key that unlocks your body's cells so that glucose can enter and be used by the cells as energy. Fat cells, particularly abdominal fat cells, lessen the sensitivity to insulin, making it harder for glucose to pass through cell walls. Because the glucose can't enter the cells, it remains in the bloodstream (high blood sugar). The pancreas responds by producing and releasing more insulin. This cycle repeats itself and grows worse over time. This is what leads to metabolic syndrome and type 2 diabetes.

Excess Belly Fat Greatly Increases the Risk of Heart Disease and Stroke

Because belly fat is so close to the liver (and often accompanied by excess fat directly surrounding the liver), it boosts production of LDL cholesterol (the one we don't want boosted!). This cholesterol eventually becomes a waxy substance known as plaque, which sticks to artery walls and eventually causes swelling, narrowing the arteries. This narrowing increases blood pressure, which seriously taxes the heart. It also increases your chance of blood clots, which can cause stroke.

Excess Belly Fat Increases the Risk of Dementia

Excess belly fat has even been linked to an increased risk of dementia. In fact, excess belly fat increases your risk of developing dementia by as much as 145%! This is a result of the same inflammation in the artery walls, which decreases proper blood flow to the brain.

With all of the serious health risks linked to belly fat, it's easy to see that getting rid of excess belly fat should be a very high priority. Fortunately, while we have lots of "scary" research that shows the risks of belly fat, we also have all of the new research that shows us how to get rid of belly fat quickly, easily and permanently.

Identifying The Two Kinds of Belly Fat

There are actually two kinds of belly fat: subcutaneous fat and visceral fat. Subcutaneous means under the skin. This is the fat you can see and pinch, since it's just below the skin layer.

Visceral fat is the fat that surrounds your vital organs. In the case of abdominal fat, your liver is most commonly affected.

Excess subcutaneous fat around the abdomen is usually accompanied by excess visceral fat around the liver.

The good news: The Belly Fat Diet plan attacks BOTH types of belly fat.

③

WHAT YOU CAN EXPECT FROM
THE BELLY FAT DIET

You Will Lose Weight, but You Will Also Specifically Lose Belly Fat

Because most diets are designed to help you lose weight by cutting and/or burning calories, they result in weight loss that includes the loss of stored water and lean muscle tissue. If you're able to stick to them for long, you may see a nice new number on the scale, but you still look flabby because you've lost muscle instead of stored fat.

This plan does not rely on simply cutting calories to lose weight. You'll probably take in fewer calories, although some people who have been on low calorie diets will actually start taking in more. The key is that you will be taking in the right calories — from foods that actually help to speed up your metabolism, burn stored fat and utilize your food better to provide energy.

You Will Not be Counting Calories, Carbs or Fat Grams

There are two reasons for this.

- This diet does not rely on cutting calories to lose belly fat.
- The foods list is designed to provide plenty of nutrition and satisfaction without empty calories, excess carbs or unhealthy fats. As long as you stick to the foods list and follow some simple guidelines, there's no need to track everything you put in your mouth.

You Will Not Be Portioning or Weighing Anything

One of the reasons that most diets fail, even diets that are based on solid science, is that they take too much time to follow correctly. People today are busy; our schedules are already overloaded and our time is already stretched too thinly. Diets that require you to keep journals, track exchanges and measure, portion and take note of every morsel are a lot like having a second job. No matter how good a diet is, if you don't have time to follow it, it won't work for you.

Again, by sticking to the foods list and following some simple guidelines, you will get plenty of food and plenty of nutrients, without getting too much fat or too many unhealthy carbs. There's nothing to track, nothing to measure.

You Will Not Be Hungry All The Time

One of the keys to losing belly fat is to eat as frequently as possible, even grazing all day long. Because of this, you won't have to be left feeling hungry or have to suffer through cravings brought on by too little food or a lack of the right nutrients.

It may take your body a week or two to get used to your new way of eating, so you may find yourself feeling hungry frequently. However, when you are hungry, you're supposed to eat! There's no need to deal with a grumbling stomach until the next scheduled meal. Eat!

You Will Not Be Tired and Grumpy

Frequent meals and snacks keep your blood sugar steady. Spikes in blood sugar are quickly followed by crashes in blood sugar. This is the cycle that occurs when you skip meals and then eat a large meal, or get too hungry and grab a snack filled with sugar and simple carbs.

This cycle will leave you feeling fatigued, foggy and irritable. It gets even worse when you limit the good carbs and fats in your diet.

The Belly Fat Diet allows you to eat whenever you want — but you're also eating a diet rich in healthy carbs and fats, so you have a steady supply of energy without all those spikes and crashes.

You Will Probably Lose Weight Faster Than You Expect

It used to be accepted as fact that you should never lose more than two pounds per week. This is because most diets cut calories to lose weight. Losing more than two pounds per week meant that you were reducing your caloric intake to unhealthy levels.

Because the Belly Fat Diet does not rely on this method, but rather helps your body to reset and maximize its fat burning and fat storing systems, you can safely lose more than two pounds per week. The old method of dieting actually caused your body to feed on itself by using its own muscle tissue as a source of protein and energy. With this plan, you'll get plenty of calories, protein and other nutrients. You'll also be resetting your body's fat burning and fat storage systems. This means that the weight you lose will be stored fat, not lean muscle, so it's perfectly safe for you to lose more than two pounds per week.

Some people might lose between five and ten pounds the first week. Do not be concerned that you're losing too much too soon. This is a response to increased metabolism, the shedding of unneeded stored water and targeting stored fat. Weight loss often then levels out in the following weeks to an average of between three and five pounds per week.

Not only will the lean muscle tissue you already have be safe, but you'll also actually be adding more lean muscle on this plan.

"It's Just Water Weight": *How many times have you heard that phrase? Fad diets do result in fast initial weight loss and a good deal of that weight is water. However, not all water weight loss is temporary. Excess sodium and processed foods cause your body's tissues to retain excess water. The Belly Fat Diet plan cuts out processed foods, additives and excess sodium, which will stimulate your body to flush out all of that unnecessary fluid. Also, the plan is a permanent lifestyle change, not a quick fix. Hopefully, you won't be going back to an unhealthy diet once you reach your fat loss goals, so you won't be packing that water back on. Therefore, some of the weight you lose in the first week or so will be water, but it won't be coming back.*

$$\left(\begin{array}{c}4\end{array}\right)$$

EVERYTHING WE THOUGHT WAS WRONG: BLASTING THE MYTHS ABOUT LOSING BELLY FAT

Until very recently, the nutrition and exercise communities had very firm ideas about losing belly fat that went back decades and seemed set in stone. It was considered scientific fact that the only way to lose belly fat was to stick to a very low-calorie, low-fat diet and spend as much time as possible (an hour or more per day was recommended) on strenuous cardio exercise and abdominal workouts.

Excess Belly Fat is *Not* Your Destiny

This long-held belief about losing belly fat led to a great deal of frustration for dieters. It supported the idea that some people were just genetically predisposed to carry more belly fat, with no hope of redesigning their bodies. Because what we were doing wasn't working, it was assumed that some of us just weren't meant to have flat abs.

The numerous research studies and findings that have come out recently offer a great deal of hope to people who had given up on ever losing that stubborn belly fat. It's much more encouraging to find out that there is a cure for excess belly fat; it just isn't what we thought it was!

Low Calorie Diets Actually Increase Belly Fat

For decades upon decades, it was accepted as simple, scientific fact that the only way to lose fat was to take in fewer calories than you use. We spent years finding our daily caloric requirements (based on sex, age, activity level and height) and figuring out how many calories we needed to cut in order to lose a pound of fat. There were a few things that made this difficult.

First, cutting calories does not specifically address losing belly fat. Second, this mathematical approach to losing weight led many people to cut their caloric intake too low. This brought about a couple of results:

- People were unable to maintain such a low-calorie diet, so they found themselves on the yo-yo dieting cycle of losing weight, falling off the diet, gaining back even more weight and starting another low-calorie diet.
- Those who were able to stay on their low-calorie diets eventually reached the infamous "weight loss plateau". This is because our metabolisms are designed to conserve energy and store fat (mostly in the abdomen) when they detect a food shortage. If your food intake is too low, your metabolism will virtually shut down to prevent starvation.

We now know that low-calorie diets are almost the opposite of what we need to lose weight, especially to lose belly fat. While you shouldn't take in twice as many calories as you can use in a day, you also shouldn't cut them too low. The balanced answer? Taking in enough (high quality) calories for your body to function efficiently and your metabolism to run at top speed.

Dietary Fat is Not the Enemy

Most of the low-calorie diets we've always been told to follow were also low-fat diets. It was assumed that all fat was bad and that we had to get it out of our diets in order to get it off of our bellies.

The problems are that *a)* fat is an essential nutrient to our bodies and *b)* without enough fat, we're unable to stick to our diets and we're back to the yo-yo cycle.

Fat not only enhances the flavor of our food, it also gives us a feeling of satisfaction and fullness, which can curb cravings and prevent overeating. Fat is also used to transport essential vitamins and minerals.

We now know that all fats are not created equal; there are bad fats, good fats and better fats.

Trans-fats, which are found in processed foods and hydrogenated oils, have no place in a healthy diet. Saturated fats, which are found primarily in animal products such as meat and butter, need to be kept to healthy levels. Polyunsaturated fats, such as olive oil, avocado and canola oil are actually good for us, as are the Omega 3 fats found in many fish, nuts and seeds.

The key is not to cut out all fat, but to cut out the bad fats and get plenty of the good ones. The healthy fats not only improve our heart health and brain function; they can also specifically help us to lose belly fat.

Burning a Ton of Calories is Not the Answer

The other long-held belief about losing belly fat was that you had to burn it off by spending hours at the gym or in a class, huffing and puffing your way to a flat belly. Again, this belief came down to math: it was thought that the more calories you burned, the more fat you lost.

Once again, this approach did not specifically target the loss of belly fat. Many people spent hours on the treadmill or in an aerobics class and saw the numbers on the scale drop while the belly fat stayed put. This is what led to the theory that some people are predisposed, by genetics and heredity, to carry more belly fat than others.

This is why we saw a surge in popular diets that claimed to work with your "set point" of weight or BMI or to address certain body types.

Thankfully, we now know that these methods and theories simply failed to address the ways and the reasons that our bodies are designed to store fat or dispose of belly fat. While our genetics and heredity may decide whether we have a long torso or wide shoulders, whether we tend to store fat on our hips or on our thighs, they do not mean that some people can have flat abs and some can't. Anyone can have a slim waist and toned abs. Some of us may have to work harder at it, but we can all achieve it.

All the Crunches in the World Won't Help You Lose Belly Fat

For years, it was accepted as fact that in order to lose belly fat, you had to do specific exercises that targeted the abs. People spent hours doing sit-ups or crunches without seeing results. There's a very simple reason for this: resistance exercise does not burn fat in a specific area. Exercise burns calories and speeds up your metabolism, but your body doesn't burn fat from your abs because you're doing crunches or burn fat from your upper arms because you're doing flies.

Cardio, and to a lesser extent, resistance exercise, burns calories overall. This can help you to lose weight overall and prevent the storage of new fat. However, this is an overall effect, not a targeted effect.

Resistance exercises such as crunches build and tone lean abdominal muscles, but your muscles are located beneath (or behind) the fat layer. This is why you can do loads of crunches and still have a fat tummy. The muscles are there, you just can't see them. In order for those crunches to result in a flat, toned tummy, you have to get rid of the fat that's hiding those muscles.

Before you get discouraged about all those wasted crunches, understand that the exercise you've been doing and the exercise you're about to do will soon pay off. If you've been working out regularly, those muscles are under there, you just need to reveal them. The Belly Fat Diet is going to help you do that, and much more quickly and easily than you're probably thinking.

Our bodies have very specific systems, checks and balances for utilizing, storing and disposing of stored fat. By using what we have learned about these processes and working with them, we can finally lose the excess belly fat that has stubbornly refused to budge.

By making some simple and even very pleasant (how does snacking all day and getting a good night's rest sound?) diet and lifestyle changes, we can finally transform our bodies into lean, toned, fat-burning machines without having to live the life of an athlete or eating the diet of a bird.

In the next section, we'll explain these fat burning and fat storing processes and how you can use them to finally get the body you've always wanted.

How to Lose Your Belly Fat

- The Top Five Tools for Losing Belly Fat Fast and Forever

- Understanding How to Break the Cortisol Cycle

- Reversing Insulin Resistance

- The Supplements That Help You Lose Belly Fat
and Feel Great Doing It

- Eating More to Weigh Less

- It's Not Cheating If It's Part of The Plan!

- The Belly Fat Diet Foods List

- Five Super-Foods You Need to Include
on Your Shopping List

- Working Out Less to Look Better Than Ever

- An Overview of Your Makeover Plan

THE TOP FIVE TOOLS FOR LOSING
BELLY FAT FAST AND FOREVER

The Belly Fat Diet takes all of the current research and all of the new findings about losing belly fat and incorporates them into one, effective and easy-to-follow plan.

The plan addresses:

- How cortisol controls the storage and disposal of belly fat and how you can break the cortisol cycle.
- How and why the hormones leptin and ghrelin can work for or against belly fat loss.
- The role insulin plays in both storing excess belly fat and regulating cravings and energy levels.
- The connection between stress and excess belly fat and how to break it.
- The role of vitamin C and Omega 3 fats in losing belly fat.
- How to boost your metabolism to burn more fat all day long.
- The most effective exercise method for losing weight and belly fat.

Tool # 1: Breaking the Cortisol Cycle

There's been so much information in the media and in diet books about the role that cortisol plays in the storage and disposal, or burning, of belly fat. If you haven't read the research or done much investigating on your own, you may not understand what cortisol is, what it does and how to break the cortisol cycle.

Cortisol is one of the stress hormones naturally produced and secreted in the body. Cortisol's specific job is to react to stress signals by storing fat in the abdominal area. The reason this system exists is because, in ages past, stress often indicated a chance of famine in the near future. Back when people moved from place to place to find food and were often considered food themselves by other predators, stress was a signal that we were on the run and food was going to be in short supply.

Very few of us are in danger of famine from the stress we're under today, but the body's system for storing fat in times of stress remains in place. To our bodies, stress is stress, whether it's from a shortage of food, a lion who thinks we look like dinner, or a boss who wants us to work long hours.

This is where the cortisol cycle comes in. We're more stressed today than people have ever been before. We have financial problems, busy schedules, demanding jobs and families to take care of in between. That stress triggers the release of cortisol into our bloodstreams, which causes our bodies to direct fat to the abdomen to be used in case of famine. The problem is, there is no famine. We continue to eat more than enough food, so that fat is never used as an energy source.

We'll tell you more in depth what you need to know about cortisol in the next few pages, but the Belly Fat Diet will break the cortisol cycle and reset your system so that your body uses dietary fat properly but also gets rid of the fat it already has stored up on your abdomen.

Tool #2: Reversing Insulin Resistance

Your hormones are at it again! Like cortisol, insulin is a hormone produced by your body, although it is not a stress hormone. The role of insulin is to regulate the amount of sugar in your bloodstream and to allow glucose (created from the foods you eat) to be used by cells as energy.

You may have heard about insulin resistance, which is a situation where your body's cells become resistant to insulin and glucose cannot pass through the cell membrane to be used as energy. When this occurs, two things happen:

- 1... your blood sugar levels spike and drop repeatedly, causing a fatigue/energy boost/fatigue cycle.
- 2... all of that unused glucose is stored as fat, mainly around your belly.

Like the situation with stress, cortisol and belly fat, insulin resistance is cyclical. The cycle goes something like this:

- Excess belly fat makes your body resistant to insulin.
- Insulin resistance causes your body to store more belly fat.
- Rinse and repeat.

This cycle is what can eventually lead to type 2 diabetes, which is why excess belly fat is a leading indicator of developing the disease. Fortunately, this cycle is reversible. In fact, *even if you already have type 2 diabetes,* losing belly fat and making the dietary changes prescribed in the Belly Fat Diet can greatly improve and even reverse the disease!

Tool #3: Vitamin C

Vitamin C has always been known as the wonder vitamin when it comes to preventing and relieving colds and other infections. However, the importance of vitamin C goes far beyond fighting infection and boosting immunity.

Vitamin C is also one of the key players in losing belly fat. It does this in two ways:

- First, vitamin C is a necessary for the production of L-carnitine, a chemical used to transport stored fat, particularly abdominal fat, to where it can be burned as energy.
- Second, vitamin C reduces the effects of stress on the body, which helps to break the cortisol cycle, so that your body is stimulated to both burn stored belly fat and to stop storing new belly fat.

Vitamin C is a soluble vitamin, which means that our bodies don't store it up in great quantities. We use a great deal of it for cell renewal and cell production and most of the rest of it is spent fighting off infection. Unfortunately, stress also uses up a great deal of vitamin C.

This means we have yet another cycle that gets in the way of losing that belly fat. We're stressed, so we have excess cortisol released into our bloodstreams, causing our bodies to store belly fat. That stress we're under also uses up all of our extra vitamin C, so there isn't enough L-carnitine to move that belly fat to where it can be repurposed as energy.

On the Belly Fat Diet plan, you'll be getting a great deal of vitamin C from your diet, which will be full of vitamin C-dense foods. But you'll also be taking a vitamin C supplement twice per day to give your body the extra C it needs to burn the belly fat you already have. This vitamin C supplementation is essential to turbo-charging the belly fat loss in the first few weeks. As an added bonus, you'll be boosting your immune system through both the vitamin C and your antioxidant-rich diet.

Tool #4: Getting Leptin and Ghrelin on Your Side

You've met cortisol; now let us introduce you to leptin and ghrelin. Both are hormones that greatly influence your weight by controlling your appetite. Leptin is secreted in fat tissue and sends a signal to your brain that lets it know you're full. Ghrelin is secreted in the intestinal tract and sends signals indicating that you're hungry.

Leptin and ghrelin aren't stress hormones, but they do have something in common with cortisol: they are impacted by your sleep habits. Several recent research studies have shown that people who get less than seven hours of sleep per night have elevated ghrelin levels and decreased leptin levels. One of the interesting findings in these studies is that one night of missed or interrupted sleep is enough to see this change in leptin and ghrelin levels. It's far more pronounced when insufficient sleep is a regular pattern, but one all-night study session or party into the wee hours is enough to interfere with the work of these two hormones.

What this means for you is that getting adequate (7-8 hours minimum) sleep, preferably at the same time each night, is essential to keeping leptin and ghrelin on your side. It won't take long to get them regulated, so that you'll soon be overeating less and seeing fewer hunger pangs. This translates to faster belly fat loss without having to do anything other than sleep!

Fish Oil Helps You Lose Belly Fat: *The DHA and EPA in Omega-3 fats have been shown to reduce symptoms of depression and signs of stress, which can help you to avoid emotional eating. Studies have also shown that people who eat plenty of oily fish and other Omega-3 rich foods lose more fat per week than dieters who don't; on average one*

pound more. The Belly Fat Diet is filled with Omega-3 fats
from fish, shellfish, avocadoes, olive oil, nuts and seeds. You'll
also be taking a fish oil supplement each day. It'll be good
for your heart, your mood and your waistline.

Tool #5: Interval Training

If you've read or heard about interval training, you may have thought it was just for athletes and those who are already pretty fit. The truth is, anyone can utilize interval training to maximize the effects of their workouts in a minimum of time.

Interval training is simply alternating periods of moderate work with shorter bursts of more intense work. You can apply it to virtually any form of exercise and you can start right where you are, even if you haven't done a bit of exercise in years. The wonderful thing is that your body reacts to the level of exertion you require for your workouts, so beginners can benefit just as much as athletes.

Interval training has been proven to be far more effective than a static (steady paced) workout. In fact, twenty minutes of interval training boosts your metabolism longer than an hour of static exercise!

Interval training works because your body adjusts itself very quickly to your workouts. As you become stronger, your metabolism works less to achieve the same number of reps or the same mileage walked. What this usually means is that people discover they have to work out longer to get the same results.

With interval training, you are constantly keeping your body guessing, so your metabolism is never given a chance to adjust and slow down.

This metabolism boost means that you'll burn more calories throughout the day, no matter what you're doing. This allows you to lose fat faster without cutting calories. Another benefit to interval training is that you don't have to spend hours working out. You can spend just twenty or thirty minutes a day on interval training. As you progress, you won't add more time to your workouts, you'll simply adjust the moderate periods to be shorter or more intense and adjust the intense periods to be longer or more difficult, still keeping your total workout time down to twenty or thirty minutes.

There's one more benefit to interval training, too. Interval training builds lean muscle faster than steady training. Lean muscle not only burns more calories than fat tissue, but it also improves the efficiency with which glucose is absorbed and burned by muscles. (Remember that glucose absorption has everything to do with reducing your risk of diabetes and losing stored belly fat.)

Conclusion

These five tools represent the best that all of the new research into fat loss and belly fat have to offer. We've taken all of them and put them into one easy-to-follow plan that will help you burn that belly fat faster than you thought possible, all while helping you to feel satisfied and energetic.

With these tools, losing that stubborn belly fat is not only possible, it's enjoyable.

6

UNDERSTANDING HOW TO BREAK
THE CORTISOL CYCLE

We've explained what cortisol is and what it does in the previous chapter. Now you need to know why cortisol is released into the bloodstream and how the Belly Fat Diet will help you to break the cortisol cycle and finally get rid of your excess belly fat quickly, painlessly and permanently.

As you read earlier, cortisol is a stress hormone. When your body perceives stress, it signals the release of cortisol into the bloodstream. That cortisol release stimulates the storage of fat around your belly, specifically on a part of your abdomen known as the omentum. The omentum is a layer of deep tissue that stretches across your abdomen behind the navel. This is why the measurement of your waist at the belly button is such an important indicator of your risk for the diseases and conditions attributed to excess belly fat.

It Doesn't Take A Lot of Stress to Stimulate Cortisol Release

This is an important fact to keep in mind. A recent study on cortisol and belly fat revealed that even the stress of counting calories increased cortisol levels in the bloodstream. While major stressors such as unemployment, the death of a loved one or divorce stimulate the release of more cortisol, the minor stressors of daily life add up to a good deal of cortisol in your bloodstream—enough to keep that belly fat growing.

The Other Factors that Stimulate Cortisol Release

The stress of everyday life and the major stressors we all encounter from time to time are not the only things that will increase cortisol production and release. Cortisol release will also be stimulated by insufficient or irregular sleep and hunger, and skipping meals.

The Belly Fat Diet addresses these factors in order to help you break the cortisol cycle. In order to reduce the amount of cortisol coursing through your system, you will:

- **Forget about counting calories, measuring grams, weighing portions or writing down everything you eat.** As we've said before, these tactics that have been so popular on other diets actually make the diets hard to stick with for any length of time. Now you know they also stress you out enough to stimulate cortisol production and keep you from losing that belly fat.

- **Get a minimum of seven hours sleep every night, on a regular schedule.** We've already explained that getting sufficient and regular sleep is essential to keeping the hormones leptin and ghrelin working for you, not against you. It's also one of the most important things you can do to break the cortisol cycle. Several research studies have been released in the last few years that investigated the link between insufficient sleep, cortisol levels and body fat ratios. All of these studies reported that people who get at least seven hours of sleep each night at fairly regular times (going to bed within the same one to two hours each night) are more likely to weight less, have smaller body fat ratios and slimmer waistlines than those who regularly sleep less than seven hours. Remember that old line about "losing weight while you sleep"? It was almost true!

- **Eat as often as possible, with no more than two hours between meals and snacks.** This one may be music to a dieter's ears, but it's based on solid, scientific research. Going more than two or three hours without eating:
  - Causes a sharp drop in blood sugar, creating cravings for unhealthy carbs and sugars.
  - Slows the metabolism.
  - Increases cortisol levels in the blood.
  - Causes fatigue and mental fogginess that has us reaching for coffee, sodas and candy bars.

On the Belly Fat Diet eating plan, you can eat anything on the foods list as often as possible without overeating or stuffing yourself. You'll also need to be sure to eat as soon after waking as you possibly can. This kick-starts your metabolism, keeps your blood sugar at a healthy level and keeps cortisol from overreacting to eight hours without food. (If you don't have the time or stomach for a full breakfast, try one of the smoothie recipes you'll find in the bonus *Belly Fat Diet Cookbook*.)

There's one other thing you can do to positively impact cortisol function: have at least fifteen minutes a day that is devoted to unwinding, loosening up, laughing and de-stressing by any means that works for you. Use a fifteen minute coffee break to get outdoors or listen to some soothing music with the office lights turned down. Play with your kids or your dog when you get home to help you detox from the little (or not so little) stresses of your day. Incorporate some yoga or yoga breathing into your workout plan. Everyone has their favorite way to let go of stress; find several of yours and use them throughout the week. If you have fifteen minutes for a phone call, surfing the web or leafing through a magazine, you have fifteen minutes to take care of yourself.

Fortunately, it doesn't take long to get your cortisol levels in line. Within a couple of weeks of starting the Belly Fat Diet, you'll have cortisol working to help you shed that belly fat.

REVERSING INSULIN RESISTANCE

As we explained previously, insulin resistance is a common result of excess belly fat. It may be a bit of a chicken-or-egg type situation as well. Insulin resistance causes excess belly fat to be stored because glucose is not being used as energy. At the same time, excess belly fat and the eating patterns that cause it can also create insulin resistance.

As with correcting the cortisol cycle, avoiding, reducing and reversing insulin resistance is achieved through dietary changes, reducing belly fat and moderate exercise. Many studies have concluded that even if you already have type 2 diabetes, you can greatly improve or even reverse it through making these lifestyle and health changes.

Fighting Insulin Resistance through Healthy Eating

The Belly Fat Diet eating plan works on correcting or preventing insulin resistance in four ways:

- Eliminating almost all processed foods, which are filled with sugar and refined flour.
- Reducing overall sugar intake.

- Increasing protein and plant fiber intake to slow absorption of carbs.
- Frequent meals and snacks to keep blood sugar steady.

Processed Foods are Not Your Friends

There are almost no processed foods allowed on the eating plan. This means no fast food, no convenience foods, no ready-made baked goods and so on. Processed foods such as these are filled with refined flours and other starches that are broken down very quickly and create a sharp increase in blood glucose levels. Your body responds with an equally sharp increase in insulin. Twenty minutes to an hour later, your blood sugar drops just as rapidly and you reach for another quick boost, usually more carbs and sugar. This cycle is credited as being one of the main causes of insulin resistance.

Carbohydrates from grains are limited on the eating plan because they're one of the easiest to overeat and among the fastest to be turned into sugar by your body's digestive system. Whole grain oatmeal and multi-grain cereals, whole grain bread and a few other high-fiber grains are allowed on the diet in limited quantities, but most of your fiber will come from plant foods, which are absorbed much more slowly.

The Eating Plan is Very Low in Added Sugar

Too much sugar in your diet presents the same problems as too much refined flour and processed food: it's absorbed very quickly into the bloodstream and wreaks havoc on your blood sugar and your insulin sensitivity.

Added sugars are allowed on the eating plan, but in much smaller quantities than many people usually eat. If at all possible, you should limit it to sweetening your coffee or tea (if you need it) and the amounts that naturally occur in allowed foods such as flavored Greek yogurts, frozen fruit bars and some of the homemade sweet treats we've included in the *Belly Fat Diet Cookbook.*

At first, you may balk at having to ration your sweets, but after a couple of weeks, your sugar cravings will be much more easily satisfied by healthier sweets such as fresh fruit, which you can eat freely on the diet.

High Protein and Fiber Intake Keeps Blood Sugar Steady

One of the other efficient ways to end the spike and drop cycle in blood sugar levels is to slow the absorption of carbs and sugars.

You may have heard or read about the glycemic index, which measures foods based on how quickly they are absorbed into the bloodstream as glucose. Examples of high-glycemic foods would be table sugar, cake, cookies and candy. Healthier foods can also have a relatively high glycemic index. Bananas rate high on the index, as do dried fruits. On the other hand, meats, eggs, cheese and vegetables such as spinach rank very low because they are converted to glucose much more slowly.

In addition to the glycemic index, there is something called the glycemic load, which is the total glycemic index of a meal or combination of foods. Some foods, when combined, create a lower glycemic load. For instance, if you have a banana by itself, its glycemic index is high, but if you have a banana with three scrambled eggs the total glycemic load is quite low.

This is because protein and fiber, when eaten with a carb food such as bread or fruit, slow the absorption of those carbs into the bloodstream. This results in a much slower rise in blood sugar after a meal, which is easily dealt with by insulin release. It also gets rid of that pesky carb crash.

On the Belly Fat Diet eating plan, you're encouraged to include a protein or high-fiber food in every meal and snack. For instance, if you feel like having an orange, we encourage you to have a mozzarella stick or boiled egg, too. This will not only lower the glycemic load of that orange, it will also keep you feeling more satisfied than if you eat the orange alone.

Frequent Meals Increase Insulin Sensitivity

As mentioned previously, frequent meals help you to reduce or avoid insulin resistance because you eliminate the blood sugar spikes and drops that come with skipping meals. You'll also be less likely to reach for forbidden snacks such as colas or candy bars to fight sluggishness. Even further, it's been shown that eating smaller, more frequent meals helps prevent overeating. Even with healthy foods, it's possible to eat too much if you let yourself get too hungry.

Improving Insulin Sensitivity through Exercise

One of the first things doctors advise patients with type 2 diabetes, metabolic syndrome or insulin resistance is to get moving. Physicians strongly urge patients who either have these issues or are at risk for them to get at least some cardiovascular (or aerobic) and resistance (or strength training) exercise each week. This is also a huge component of the Belly Fat Diet.

The ways that exercise improves insulin sensitivity can get a little complicated and explaining them can get a little too technical, so we'll break it down into a somewhat oversimplified, two-step process.

Let's start with the two types of effects that exercise has on insulin sensitivity. They're known as the acute (or immediate and temporary) effect and the training (long term) effect. Studies have shown conclusively that even a single bout of moderate exercise improves insulin sensitivity for a short period of time; anywhere from twelve hours to two days. This is the acute effect. These same studies show that regular, moderate exercise soon results in a round-the-clock improvement in insulin sensitivity. This is known as the training effect.

Moderate cardiovascular exercise, such as twenty to thirty minutes of walking, biking, swimming or dancing, is enough for your body reap the benefits of increased insulin sensitivity.

The same is true of resistance training. However, resistance training offers some extra benefits.

When you train your muscles, they use glycogen (the form of glucose that is stored in muscle and used as energy) to both provide energy and rebuild muscle tissue. They also continue to "request" glucose for up to 24 hours after the workout. This means that there's less glucose roaming around in your bloodstream and less insulin needed to deal with it. That is the acute effect of resistance training.

However, there are actually two types of training effects created by resistance or strength training. First, regular strength training produces the training effect that we've already discussed. Second, the more lean muscle you have, the more efficiently your body uses glucose and insulin overall. Fat tissue doesn't need glucose, it stores it. Muscle tissue uses glucose for energy. The more lean muscle you have, the more glucose you need and the less glucose you have being added to fat stores, especially around your tummy.

We'll provide more detail and several workout plans in the exercise section, but the Belly Fat Diet includes twenty to thirty minutes of cardio exercise at least three times per week and twenty to thirty minutes of resistance training at least three times per week. That's enough to get your insulin sensitivity back to maximum performance and help you to Belly Fat Diet and build a leaner, stronger body.

Many people report noticing a change in their energy levels, mood, cravings and hunger (signs of improved insulin sensitivity) almost immediately, but expect it to take a couple of weeks for you to see a real difference.

Note: *You should talk to your doctor before starting any diet or exercise program, but if you've been diagnosed with type 2 diabetes, it is particularly essential that you let your doctor know your plans (for both diet and exercise) before you get started.*

(8)

THE SUPPLEMENTS THAT HELP YOU TO LOSE BELLY FAT AND FEEL GREAT WHILE YOU'RE DOING IT

While the Belly Fat Diet eating plan is filled with foods that are packed with vitamins, minerals, antioxidants and other essential micronutrients, you'll also be taking a few select supplements that will further nourish your body and help you to lose that belly fat.

It's best to get your doctor's okay before starting on a supplement program, so do discuss the list with your doctor before you begin. In some cases, current health issues and regular medications may require some adjustment.

The Daily Supplement Plan

Each morning and evening (or late afternoon), you'll be taking:

- 1000mg vitamin C (chewable tablets are fine)
- 1000mg of a high-quality fish oil supplement
- 1 B-Vitamin Complex (ask your doctor for recommended dosage)

We've already discussed vitamin C at length and its importance in reducing cortisol and producing L-Carnitine to transport stored fat. Because vitamin C is a soluble vitamin, our bodies don't store much; any excess will be disposed of as waste, so there's no need to worry about taking too much unless if you get into mega-dosing (amounts ranging from 5,000 to 10,000 daily).

The fish oil supplement is an added dose of healthy Omega-3 fats to supplement those you're getting through your diet. Be sure to read the labels and even ask for help at the health food store or pharmacy where you purchase it. You want a supplement that contains both DHA and EPA. If you really don't care for fish and seafood, you may want to ask your doctor about increasing the amount of fish oil you take daily, as you'll be getting less of it through your diet.

The B-complex of vitamins are also soluble vitamins. Since our bodies don't store them in any real quantity, most of our supply has to come through our daily diet. The fruits and vegetables you'll be eating will provide a healthy supply, but taking a supplement insures that your immune system and energy levels are getting all they need.

EATING MORE TO WEIGH LESS

The Belly Fat Diet eating plan allows you to eat as much of the allowed foods as you want, as often as possible. This will keep hunger and cravings at bay, keep your energy high, your blood sugar steady and just make you a whole lot happier and more willing to stick with the plan.

However, there are some guidelines to follow.

Eating as Much as You Want Does Not Mean Loading Up Your Plate

Unless you're piling raw veggies on your plate, you need to use some common sense about how much to eat at once.

Part of reshaping the way you eat is helping your body to be happy with "just enough" food. This means that if you're having chicken breast, a salad and a baked sweet potato for dinner, you should eat slowly and finish everything before deciding you want more. If you are still hungry, by all means, have another breast or some more veggies. However, your goal should be to eat just until satisfied, not until stuffed. Overstuffing your digestive system is counterproductive to your goals and makes you feel sluggish and uncomfortable.

Did you know? *It really does take about 20 minutes for your body to register the food you're eating. For meals, make sure you take at least twenty minutes to eat. Then decide if you're still hungry.*

Learn to Read Your Hunger

As your body adjusts to a healthier diet and your hormones begin to cooperate with you, you'll experience fewer cravings, especially for sweets. This usually takes about two weeks. However, you'll have those times when you're hungry, especially in the first few weeks. It's perfectly okay to eat, but for those times when you're standing in front of the fridge, unsure of what it is you want, try satisfying yourself with these foods in this order:

- Try some water — thirst often masks itself as hunger.
- If you're still hungry or just know you crave actual chewing, try a vegetable.
- If you're still hungry, try a fruit.
- If you're still hungry, go for a protein.
- (You get grains in such limited quantities; don't waste them on a random nosh.)

Why is this order important? For those times when you know you're not truly hungry but are just bored or need something to crunch or chew, trying these foods in this order will keep you from reaching for the higher calorie, higher fat and higher carbs foods first and eating more than you need to satisfy an urge that isn't really hunger-based.

This is not the same situation as planned snacks and meals. This is for eating out of boredom, stress or nervousness, or what is commonly called emotional eating.

Your Three Limitations: Beef, Sweet Treats and Grains

There are only three food categories that carry some limitations. They are beef, grains and sweet treats.

Beef is limited because it typically contains a good deal of unhealthy fats, is expensive to buy in healthier, grass-fed varieties and is usually eaten in fairly large portions. You're limited to one serving per week of steak or roast; the leaner cut the better, trimmed of visible fat. If you don't eat beef, that's all the better. If you truly love it and doing without it every day is going to be a challenge, reward yourself with your favorite steak once a week.

Most grains are limited because they are easy to overeat, quickly converted to sugar or glucose and many of them fail to fill you up for very long. You're limited to two servings per day of the grains on the allowed foods list.

Sweet treats are allowed on the eating plan, but they're limited to one per day and only the sweet treats that are on the allowed foods list. These are few, but tasty. They include frozen fruit pops, nonfat pudding, sorbet and dark chocolate. Use moderation is your servings of these foods and try to really enjoy them. Eat them at a time when you can focus on how good they taste, rather than eating them mindlessly or in a rush.

(10)

IT'S NOT CHEATING
IF IT'S PART OF THE PLAN!

N ow that you've heard about the few limitations and rules of the eating plan, it's time to let you in on one guideline that will probably be quite welcome. You're supposed to cheat.

Once a week, you are allowed to have one thing that you've been craving, missing, waiting for and doing without. If your true love is pizza, have it. If you've been going through milkshake withdrawal, get one.

Of course, you need to use a bit of sense here. You're not supposed to have a whole pizza, but a slice or two. If you can make it a thin crust veggie pizza, that would be awesome, but if Hawaiian with extra cheese is the only thing that makes you happy, have it. Any kind, with any of the enemies you feel like loading on top of it — but just have one or two slices.

If you've been waiting all week for Fettuccine Alfredo, then you deserve to really enjoy it ... a sensible portion of it.

If you've been dying for a Snickers, some dinner rolls and some chips, we're afraid you're going to have to pick one. The others can be your cheat for next week.

Some Guidelines to Help You Cheat the Right Way

Aside from the One Cheat Once Per Week rule and the caution about portions, there are a few tips and guidelines that can help you cheat the right way.

If you're longing for a few different foods, try to choose the one that is either the healthiest or highest in protein.

If one coveted food has sugar and the other doesn't, opt for the one without sugar. It'll affect insulin and blood sugar less.

Try to choose foods you really love, rather than wasting your weekly cheat on something that just shows up. In other words, don't give in to an unplanned slice of mediocre cake at an office party when you've been looking forward to having gourmet ice cream on Saturday.

Why You're Supposed to Cheat

The answer to this may seem obvious, but it bears explaining anyway. There are actually a few reasons why it's a good idea to plan a controlled, weekly cheat.

Knowing you're going to have that gourmet ice cream Saturday makes it easier to do without your usual nightly bowl.

Going without your favorite foods indefinitely leads to frustration, resentment and out-of-control cheating. Limiting yourself to your daily sweet and a weekly cheat takes some getting used to at first, but it's much easier than going without altogether. This means you have a much better chance of sticking to the plan until you've reached your goals....and being happier while you do.

Eventually, you'll reach your fat loss goals and be ready to move on to a more lenient diet. However, you need to have healthy habits in place when you do or you'll be right back where you started before too long. Putting off indulgences and using some sense when indulging are habits that have to be learned, but they'll serve you well later on.

Truthfully, life is hard enough. No bread lover should have to live without yeast rolls forever. You're working hard at changing your health and your body. You deserve a weekly cheat and if done right, it won't undo any of that hard work.

THE BELLY FAT DIET FOODS LIST

I n the included *Belly Fat Diet Shopping Guide,* you'll find a much more detailed list of the foods you're allowed to eat on the Belly Fat Diet eating plan. You may want to make several copies and circle items as you plan your menus and your grocery shopping.

Here, we'll give you an overview of what you'll be eating.

Meat and Poultry

You're free to eat chicken breast or ground chicken breast, turkey breast or ground turkey breast and eggs as often as you like. If you want to make sandwiches or salads with these meats, please use leftover home cooked poultry rather than packaged or deli counter meats. Those contain far too much sodium and too many nitrates and preservatives.

You're allowed lean cuts of beef steak or beef roast once a week.

Fish and Seafood

You can have as much fish and seafood as you like, as long as it isn't breaded, fried or covered in a cream sauce. It should be steamed, broiled, baked, boiled or sautéed in a bit of olive or canola oil.

Try to focus on oily, cold water fish, as they're the richest in Omega-3 fats. On the foods list, we've listed those varieties for you. However, you're free to eat any variety you like.

Dairy Products

Dairy products are limited to skim or reduced fat milk, low-fat or nonfat mozzarella and cottage cheese and Greek yogurt. (Greek yogurt has twice the protein of regular yogurt so it has more staying power and balances out the sugar.)

Try to limit the milk to using for coffee, cereal and cooking, rather than using it as a beverage. Milk is actually a food, not a drink. This will keep your intake down to a healthy level. However, if a cold glass of milk is a real treat for you, go ahead and have it, just keep it down to one glass a day.

Butter and butter substitutes are off-limits, as are other cheeses.

Fruits and Vegetables

You can have any fruit you like, as often as you like. Fresh is best, but frozen fruits (without syrup or added sugar) are fine for out-of-season fruits or for adding to smoothies and other treats. When using fruit as a snack, try to couple it with a protein to lessen the effect on your blood sugar. For example, if you're in the mood for some grapes, have them with a stick of mozzarella or a boiled egg.

All vegetables are allowed on the plan, with the exception of white potatoes and corn. Both are high in starch, which means they're quickly converted to sugar.

Veggies are best eaten raw, but steaming, roasting, baking, sautéing and stir-frying are perfectly fine. As with fruits, fresh veggies are best but frozen vegetables without butter sauce or cheese sauce added are perfectly acceptable.

Canned fruits and veggies are off limits, as they usually contain fewer vitamins and minerals, less fiber and a good deal of sugar and additives.

Grains

Grains are a good source of fiber, but most of them are converted to sugar quite quickly. They're also one of the easiest foods to overeat. For this reason, grains are limited to two servings per day and you may choose from whole-wheat, whole grain breads and cereals, brown rice, quinoa, barley and whole grain oats.

When you're choosing your grains, it's a good idea to opt for the most filling choice. A slice of whole grain toast won't stick with you for long, but a bowl of mixed-grain hot cereal will.

Nuts, Seeds and Oils

Nuts and seeds can be an excellent source of healthy fats and fiber, as long as you eat the right ones. Walnuts and almonds are your best choice and should be eaten either raw or roasted without salt or sugar. You may also have almond butter or sesame butter that has no trans-fats or sugar added. Avocadoes, olive oil and canola oil are also allowed, as well as pumpkin, sesame and poppy seeds.

Condiments and Sweet Treats

Refer to the included *Belly Fat Diet Shopping Guide* for a more detailed list, but condiments that are not packed with sugars and unhealthy fats are allowed. Ketchup, mayonnaise and Miracle Whip are off limits.

You've already heard about the sweet treats that you can choose from daily, but to repeat, they include frozen fruit pops with no added sugar, sorbets without added sugar, nonfat pudding (the sugared variety, rather than artificially sweetened — no artificial sweeteners are allowed on the plan) and dark chocolate. Limit yourself to one pop, one pudding cup, one scoop of sorbet and one piece of chocolate the size of a dental floss box.

Beverages

Beverages are limited to water, coffee, green tea and black tea. You can sweeten your coffee and tea if you must, but limit the sugar in the rest of your diet to accommodate. Black coffee is better than coffee with milk, but milk is allowed while artificial and flavored creamers are not.

You need to drink a minimum of 64 ounces of plain water per day, more if you spend a good deal of time outdoors.

Juices are not on the diet because they contain little or no fiber, don't fill you up like the whole fruit will and are easy to overdo. The same is true of flavored waters. Sodas are strictly off limits. Save them for your cheat day if you're really attached to your colas.

Other allowed foods include unsweetened protein powder, honey, agave nectar (as a sugar substitute) all herbs and seasonings and a few other items that will make it easier for you to plan delicious and nutritious meals. The grocery list in the *Belly Fat Diet Shopping Guide* will give you a more complete rundown of what's allowed.

$$\left(\,12\,\right)$$

FIVE SUPER-FOODS YOU NEED TO INCLUDE ON YOUR SHOPPING LIST

All of the foods included on the Belly Fat Diet are extremely healthy and taste great to boot. However, there are some real superstars in the food world: foods that have become known as "super-foods" in the nutritional community.

There are a number of foods that have been given their fifteen minutes of well-deserved fame recently. These include berries, soybeans and soy products, acai and many others. They're all nutritional winners, but no single food will give you everything you need. A variety of these extremely valuable foods is what you need to see a drastic change in how you look and feel.

We've highlighted five stars that are easily found in your local store, very affordable and generally well-liked by most people. Keep these on your running grocery list and eat at least one of them each day to give your immune system an extra boost.

Berries

Berries are loaded with vitamin C and several of the B-vitamins. They're also packed with phytonutrients and antioxidants. The darker the color, the better they are for you. Cranberries, black raspberries, blueberries and blackberries are all excellent choices.

Salmon

Salmon is one of the best fish choices for getting Omega-3 fatty acids. If salmon is too rich for either your taste buds or your budget, sardines, mackerel, tuna, cod and other cold water fish are equally good, but more affordable choices.

Nuts

Nuts have gotten a bad rap, mostly because people don't understand the difference between healthy fats and unhealthy ones, but also because many of us tend to indulge in varieties that aren't that great for you, such as macadamias and cashews. Nuts provide protein, heart-healthy fats, a ton of insoluble fiber and a bonus dose of antioxidants. Walnuts and almonds are your healthier choices and you should eat them in as natural a state as possible. Raw is best, roasted okay, too, as long as you skip the salted or honey-roasted types.

Kiwi

Kiwi is a nutritional jackpot, but also one of the most affordable super-foods around. Sometimes available for as little a dime each, these tasty gems are a nutritional bargain. They're packed with vitamin C and fiber, and have few calories.

Sweet Potatoes

These delicious and nutritious vegetables are one of the many orange veggies that make the various super-foods lists. They're very cheap, are packed with antioxidants, have a good amount of protein and are high in fiber. They also contain a healthy dose of Vitamin C. One of the nice things about sweet potatoes is that they satisfy the sweet tooth, too. Roast or bake them and flavor with a bit of olive oil, salt and pepper and you'll never miss the butter or that less-healthy white baked potato you used to eat.

There are many other foods we could include on this list, but adding just these five to your daily diet every week will have a terrific impact on your health, energy level and how much you enjoy your new eating lifestyle.

$$\left(\boxed{13}\right)$$

WORKING OUT LESS TO LOOK
BETTER THAN EVER

G etting regular exercise, through both cardio exercise and resistance/ strength training, is an integral part of losing belly fat. It burns calories, speeds up your metabolism, helps your body to use glucose and regulate insulin and reshapes your body.

The workout program included in the Belly Fat Diet is customizable to you and your preferences, can be done by anyone at any level of fitness, requires only a few pieces of optional, inexpensive equipment and can be done in thirty minutes per day.

Interval Training Basics

As you read earlier, interval training is simply the alternating of moderate work with more intense work. You can use interval training for virtually any cardio exercise, including walking, running, swimming, biking or dancing. With walking and running you can increase the intensity by changing the terrain or increasing speed. With swimming, you can do the crawl for your moderate periods and the butterfly for your intense periods or simply increase your speed. You get the idea.

Interval training is also easily incorporated into strength training or resistance training. You simply alternate a strength training move, such as three sets of biceps curls, with one minute of running on the treadmill, jumping rope or jumping jacks. Any cardio exercise will do, even dancing to your favorite fast song.

Here are some guidelines to keep in mind about interval training:

1. Always warm up for two minutes, whether you're doing cardio or strength training.

2. Always cool down for two minutes by stretching.

3. Always begin and end with a moderately paced segment.

4. Moderately paced segments should be longer than your intense segments. You can adjust the length of each period to suit your fitness level, but it should still remain about 2:1. In other words, the moderate segment should be twice as long as the intense segment. If you walk at a moderate pace for four minutes, you walk uphill or at a faster pace for two, and so on.

An Overview of the Workout Program

You're going to be able to customize your workouts to meet your needs, likes and fitness level. We provide several options in the next section, but here are the basics.

The goal is to work out for thirty minutes a day, six days a week. You can divide this schedule in a couple of different ways.

Six days a week, you can do the 50/50 Combo Blast, which is fifteen minutes of cardio and fifteen minutes of strength training in one workout. You'd do the same cardio routine each day and alternate the lower body and upper body strength training sessions. That would look something like this:

- Monday, Wednesday, Friday: 50/50 Lower Body Combo
- Tuesday, Thursday, Saturday: 50/50 Upper Body Combo

Or,

Three days a week you can do one of the cardio workouts and three days a week you can do one of the whole body strength training workouts. So:

- Monday, Wednesday, Friday: 30 Minute Cardio Workout
- Tuesday, Thursday, Saturday: 30 Minute Strength Training Workout

This workout plan is supposed to be fun, varied and interesting, so feel free to do the *50/50 Workouts* for a month and then switch to the *30 Minute Workouts.* You can also use walking for your cardio one month and switch to swimming the next. It's best to stick with one plan for a month so that you can properly track your progress and set new goals, but there's nothing wrong with switching it out every month. In fact, it will keep your body guessing and help you avoid that dreaded plateau while you're warding off boredom.

Customizing Your Workouts and Changing Your Workouts as You Progress

Cardio Workouts: We provide several suggested cardio workouts in the next section, but once you feel comfortable with the guidelines, you're free to come up with other ways of getting your cardio. The only caveat is that it be something that you can integrate with interval training easily. Basketball is great exercise, but not necessarily a good candidate for interval training. Rollerblading is, as are rowing, dancing and many other great forms of cardio.

Strength Training: Stick to the suggested routines until you know what you're doing. To make them accessible and affordable to everyone, we've made our routines easy to do at home without expensive equipment. If you want to switch to using a gym later on, or if you already have or want to buy a weight machine or treadmill, you're certainly encouraged to do so.

With cardio, consistency and endurance are more important than speed, so please start off slowly and safely. Interval training allows you to progress more quickly than static training, so you're going to make progress soon enough. If you hurt yourself or become discouraged by starting off at a level that is too difficult for you, you'll sabotage yourself and derail your efforts.

With strength training, maintaining proper form is far more important than the amount of weight you lift or number of reps and sets you do. Again, start off at a level that is appropriate to your fitness level. Our strength training workouts all use your body weight as resistance. If you like, you can add a resistance band or dumbbell workout later. When you do, you should only lift as much weight as you can lift with perfect form. The last rep should be hard, but if you're in danger of dropping the weight, you're lifting too much.

You're going to see dramatic results from interval training in a very short period of time. Be patient, be safe and have fun.

AN OVERVIEW OF YOUR MAKEOVER PLAN

Now that you know the components of the Belly Fat Diet, let's put it all together in one easy-to-follow list, so that you can refer to it as needed without having to page through the entire book.

The Eating Plan:

- Eat only the foods on the foods list.
- Eat as often as possible, with no more than three hours between meals or snacks. Two is better. You can eat three main meals and unlimited snacks or just eat several mini-meals and snacks all day, whichever suits your lifestyle and personality.
- Eat as soon after waking as you can, even if it's just a snack.
- Eat one sweet treat per day. You can skip it if you don't care for sweets, but you can't have more than one per day.
- Once a week, you'll have a planned cheat, according to the guidelines.
- Take the recommended supplements twice per day, every day.

The Workout Plan:

- Target working out for 30 minutes, six days a week, using either the 50/50 Combo Workouts or alternating the 30 Minute Workouts.

Also:

- Try to sleep at least seven hours per night at roughly the same time each night, ideally going to bed within the same two hour time period every night.
- You want to drink a minimum of 64 ounces of water per day.

Putting the Belly Fat Diet Into Action

- Two Examples for Your Meal Plans

- Tips for Planning Your Meals

- Introduction to the Workout Plans

- The 50/50 Workout Plans

- The 30 Minute Workout Plans

TWO EXAMPLES FOR YOUR MEAL PLANS

The Belly Fat Diet Plan is supposed to allow you some freedom of choice in your diet, as well as a simple to follow plan. How you divide your meals is up to your preferences, your lifestyle and your schedule. If you want to graze all day, without planning regular, larger meals, you can do that. If you want to plan three regular meals with several snacks in between, you can do that, too.

Here are a couple of examples that can help you map out the meal plan that works best for you.

A Grazing Plan

(The times are just examples we're using instead of meals)

8am: Dr. Oz's Smoothie or the Sunshine Smoothie (recipe in the included *Belly Fat Diet Cookbook*)

10am: An apple and a cheese stick

12pm: Boiled egg, spinach and tomato wrap with vinaigrette

2pm: Greek yogurt and red grapes

4pm: Coffee, celery sticks with almond butter

6pm: Chicken breast and brown rice soup

8pm: Dark chocolate and an orange

10pm: Green tea and cottage cheese with fresh peaches

A Traditional Meal Plan:

Breakfast:

- Scrambled eggs with mushrooms, peppers and onion
- Slice of whole grain toast with almond butter
- Sliced apple
- Coffee

Morning Snack:

- Cheese stick and an orange

Late Morning Snack:

- Grapes and almonds

Lunch:

- Chicken soup
- Boiled egg
- Pineapple spears

Afternoon Snack:

- Sesame butter and honey on a slice of whole-grain bread

Dinner:

- Broiled salmon
- Sautéed spinach, shallots and mushrooms
- Baked sweet potato
- Salad with romaine, red peppers, onion and honey-lime dressing

Evening Snack:

- Two slices of watermelon

Late Night Snack:

- Greek yogurt

As you can see, you can divide up your food any way you like, plan as much or as little as you prefer and eat as often as you want. Feel free to mix and match days as well, to suit a changing schedule or just to keep things interesting.

The only things you need to do are stick to the foods list and the guidelines.

(16)

TIPS FOR PLANNING YOUR MEALS

Planning meals on a diet can be a real chore. If you try the following tips, however, you might find it's easier than you think!

- ***If you have limited time to cook, you can double the time you do have by doubling the recipe.*** Instead of roasting one chicken, roast two. Serve one tonight and use the other for sandwiches, salads and soups throughout the week. Instead of baking two sweet potatoes for your dinner, bake four and take the leftovers to work for a quick snack. Instead of making six cups of soup, make twelve and freeze the extra in small containers.

- ***Each weekend, put together a stash of quick snacks for the office.*** Load up a lunch bag or tote with your favorite fruits, nuts, cheese sticks, yogurts and containers of soup and other standbys and stick it in the fridge until Monday morning. This way, you always have snacks handy and can stick to your diet even when you forget your lunch. It takes a lot less time than packing snacks each morning, too.

- ***Keep an inexpensive blender at work***, as well as your favorite protein powder, a small container of milk or almond milk, and a few Ziploc bags of frozen fruit. You'll be able to grab a smoothie when hunger hits or you don't have time for lunch.

- ***Try a few new foods each week.*** They can either be exotic fruits you've never tasted, types of fish you never knew heard of or just foods you rarely remember to buy. Varying your diet not only keeps it interesting, it also ensures a wide variety of nutrients.

- ***Anticipate cooking challenges.*** Dieting when you have a family or spouse who isn't joining you can present a tough test of your diet commitment. Don't worry! Many delicious meals can be adapted to the Belly Fat Diet Diet without your loved ones noticing. You can also modify your portion of a meal so that it meets the guidelines. For instance, if you're making barbecued chicken breasts for the kids, just roast yours without sauce. If your husband is having pork chops, sweet potatoes, green beans and a salad, skip the chops, load up on the veggies and heat up a slice of turkey for your plate. The point is to avoid cooking two separate meals: one for you and one for everyone else. It saves time and energy better spent elsewhere and can also avoid making you feel frustrated and isolated.

INTRODUCTION TO THE WORKOUT PLANS

A Note for Beginners

These workouts are designed so that anyone can do them, without any equipment other than a good pair of shoes. However, if you are completely new to working out and need instruction for specific stretches and the weight training moves, there are plenty of books and DVDs that can help. Better yet, get free help on the internet. Sparkpeople.com, Shape.com and FitnessMagazine.com are all excellent resources for free slide shows and short instruction videos of each move.

Kicking it Up

As you gain strength and endurance, you'll want to kick things up a bit. Do this at your pace and forget about what your friend, spouse or co-worker is doing. Your plan is about you.

To increase the intensity of your cardio workouts, you can simply shorten your moderate segments and lengthen your intense segments, add rougher terrain or even add small dumbbells to a walking workout.

To increase the intensity of your weight training, you can do more reps in the same time, add a resistance band or dumbbells or start using a weight machine. Again, you can find plenty of free videos online that will show you how to do this.

⑱

THE 50/50 WORKOUT PLANS

The 50/50 Workout Plans incorporate both cardio and strength training into a 30 minute workout. You'll do the same cardio workout each day, six days a week, choosing from the walking, running, biking or swimming plans.

You'll do the lower body strength training routine and the upper body strength training routine on alternate days. (Both of these include some abdominal exercises, since you can safely and effectively work your abs without a day of rest in between sessions.)

Your cardio workouts take 20 minutes and your strength training takes 10.

When you're doing the 50/50 Workout Plans, it's best to start with your cardio. Your resistance training workout goal is muscle fatigue. That's what builds lean muscle fast, but it isn't a good idea to exhaust your muscles right before you head out for a run.

If you're doing your cardio outdoors and strength training at home, don't worry about the downtime in between. Contrary to traditional thought, you don't need do thirty minutes of uninterrupted exercise to reap the benefits; you just need to do the thirty minutes. Of course, if you're raring to go, you can choose an indoor cardio workout so that you can move right on to the strength training.

Cardio

Cardio Workout for Walking Outdoors

2 Minutes: Stretching and warm up — be sure to stretch your neck, shoulders, arms, back and legs.

4 Minutes: Walk at a moderate pace.

2 Minutes: Walk at a fast pace, fast enough to prevent easy conversation.

4 Minutes: Walk at a moderate pace.

2 Minutes: Walk at a fast pace.

4 Minutes: Walk at a moderate pace.

2 Minutes: Cool down by repeating your stretching exercises.

Cardio Workout for Walking or Running on a Treadmill

2 Minutes: Stretching and warm up.

4 Minutes: Walk/run at a moderate pace or on a flat terrain.

2 Minutes: Walk/run at a fast pace or on an incline

4 Minutes: Walk/run at a moderate pace or flat terrain.

2 Minutes: Walk/run at a fast pace or on an incline.

4 Minutes: Walk/run at a moderate pace or on a flat terrain.

2 Minutes: Cool down by repeating your stretching exercises.

Cardio Workout for Running Outdoors

(Recommended only for those already accustomed to running regularly)

2 Minutes: Stretching and warm up.

4 Minutes: Run at a moderate pace on a flat terrain.

2 Minutes: Run sprints or up and down stairs.

4 Minutes: Run at a moderate pace.

2 Minutes: Run sprints or up and down stairs.

4 Minutes: Run at a moderate pace.

2 Minutes: Cool down by repeating stretching exercises.

Cardio Workout for Cycling (Indoors or Outdoors)

2 Minutes: Stretching and warm up.

4 Minutes: Cycle at a moderate pace or low resistance.

2 Minutes: Cycle at a fast pace or higher resistance.

4 Minutes: Cycle at a moderate pace or low resistance.

2 Minutes: Cycle at a fast pace or higher resistance.

4 Minutes: Cycle at a moderate pace or low resistance.

2 Minutes: Cool down by repeating stretching exercises.

Cardio Workout for Swimming

2 Minutes: Stretching and warm up (in or out of the water).

4 Minutes: Swim at a moderate pace using the crawl stroke.

2 Minutes: Swim at a faster pace or using the butterfly stroke.

4 Minutes: Swim at a moderate pace using the crawl stroke.

2 Minutes: Swim at a faster pace or using the butterfly stroke.

4 Minutes: Swim at a moderate pace using the crawl stroke.

2 Minutes: Cool down by repeating stretching exercises.

Lower Body Strength Training Routine

1 Minute: Warm up by stretching.

Do twenty front lunges, five for each leg.

1 Minute: Run in place, jump rope or do jumping jacks.

Do ten squats.

1 Minute: Run in place, jump rope, or do jumping jacks.

Do twenty hamstring lifts (aka toe raises).

1 Minute: Run in place, jump rope or do jumping jacks.

Do twenty leg lifts or reverse crunches.

1 Minute: Run in place, jump rope or do jumping jacks.

Do twenty modified crunches. (Lifting only until shoulders leave the floor.)

1 Minute: Cool down by repeating stretching exercises.

Upper Body Strength Training Routine

1 Minute: Warm up by stretching.

Do twenty push-ups. If full body pushups are too difficult, start on your knees with ankles crossed.

1 Minute: Same cardio as above.

Do twenty seated chair dips.

1 Minute: Same cardio as above.

Do twenty alternating crunches (aka oblique or scissor crunches).

1 Minute: Same cardio as above.

1 Minute: Cool down by repeating stretching exercises.

THE 30 MINUTE WORKOUT PLANS

The 30 Minute Workout Plans use the same moves and steps as the 50/50 Plans. You're simply combining workouts and doing them on alternating days. Three days per week, say Mon-Wed-Fri, you'll do your cardio workout. The other three days, Tues/Thurs/Sat, you'll do a combined strength training workout. Feel free to switch these days around, they're just an example.

The 30 Minute Cardio Workout

To do the 30 Minute Cardio Workout, simply choose your preferred method of cardio from the 50/50 Plans and double the number of segments, with the exception of the warm up and cool down times.

The 30 Minute Strength Training Workout

2 Minutes: Warm up by stretching.

Do twenty front lunges, five for each leg.

1 Minute: Run in place, jump rope or do jumping jacks.

Do ten squats.

1 Minute: Same cardio as above.

Do twenty hamstring lifts (aka toe raises).

1 Minute: Same cardio as above.

Do twenty leg lifts or reverse crunches.

1 Minute: Same cardio as above.

Do twenty modified crunches. (Lifting only until shoulders leave the floor.)

1 Minute: Same cardio as above.

Do twenty alternating crunches (aka oblique or scissor crunches).

1 Minute: Same cardio as above.

Do twenty push-ups. If full body pushups are too difficult, start on your knees with ankles crossed.

1 Minute: Same cardio as above.

Do twenty seated chair dips.

1 Minute: Same cardio as above.

2 Minutes: Cool down by repeating stretching exercises.

Thanks for reading *The Belly Fat Diet*!

Any questions or comments? We'd love to hear your feedback! Please don't hesitate to send us an email at:

info@rockridgeuniversity.com

Thanks,

John Chatham and the team at Rockridge University Press

The
Belly Fat Diet

The Cookbook

Breakfast Recipes

Ranchero Roll Ups

Beat eggs and sauté in oil. When eggs are almost set add green onions.	2 eggs
	1 green onion, sliced
	3 tablespoons salsa
Wrap tortillas in damp paper towel and heat in microwave for 15 to 30 seconds. Place half of the egg on each tortilla, add salsa and roll up to serve.	1 teaspoon canola oil
	2 whole grain tortillas

"Dr. Oz" Protein Smoothie – No. 1

Put all ingredients into blender and mix until frothy.	1 scoop chocolate soy protein powder
	½ banana
	½ teaspoon flax seed
	1 teaspoon psyllium husk
	8 oz. water

"Dr. Oz" Protein Smoothie – No. 2

Put all ingredients into blender and mix until frothy.	1 scoop vanilla soy protein powder
	½ teaspoon flax seed
	1 teaspoon psyllium husk
	1 tablespoon honey
	¼ cup frozen blueberries
	8 oz. water

Sunrise Smoothie

Put all ingredients into blender and mix until frothy.	½ cup orange juice
	½ cup pineapple juice
	½ cup sliced mango
	½ banana
	1 scoop vanilla soy protein powder

Green Smoothie

Put all ingredients into blender and mix until frothy.	1 cucumber, peeled and sliced
	½ lemon, juiced
	½ cup parsley
	1 stalk celery, sliced
	½ cup plain Greek yogurt
	½ cup cold water

Summary Fruit Salad

Mix fruit in a large bowl. Store in a covered plastic container in refrigerator. Serve with cottage cheese or Greek yogurt if desired.	1 cantaloupe, sliced, peeled and cut in 1 inch pieces 1 cup fresh pineapple chunks 2 kiwi fruit, peeled, sliced and halved 1 pint blueberries, washed and sorted 1 cup seedless grapes, washed

Winter Fruit Compote

Combine all ingredients in a saucepan and bring just to a boil over medium heat. Remove from heat, cool and store in covered container in refrigerator. Serve warm with oatmeal or granola.	½ cup dried cherries ½ cup dried blueberries 12 dried apricots 1½ cups freshly pressed apple juice (chop, put in blender, strain) 1 tablespoon lemon juice ½ teaspoon cinnamon ½ teaspoon allspice

Crunchy Granola

Preheat oven to 350 degrees.

In a small bowl, mix the oil, orange juice and honey together. In a large bowl mix together the remaining ingredients until well combined. Drizzle the oil mixture over the dry ingredients and stir until evenly coated. Pack the mixture tightly into a 9 × 13 inch glass baking dish and bake for 30 minutes until golden brown. Let cool completely then break into chunks and store in an airtight container. Serve with hot or cold low-fat milk or almond milk as a cereal.

2 tablespoons canola oil

¼ cup freshly squeezed orange juice

¼ cup honey

1 cup oats

1 cup raw almonds

1 cup raw walnuts

¼ cup sesame seeds

¼ cup flax seeds

1 teaspoon ground cinnamon

½ teaspoon nutmeg

½ teaspoon powdered ginger

½ teaspoon sea salt

1 tablespoon orange zest

Egg Muffins

Whisk eggs, salt and pepper and cook in olive oil over medium heat. Stir in the onion and red pepper before eggs are set. Serve on muffins.

3 eggs

2 green onions, sliced thin

¼ cup sweet red pepper, sliced thin

½ teaspoon sea salt

¼ teaspoon cayenne pepper

1 teaspoon extra virgin olive oil

2 whole grain English muffins, toasted

Turkey Hash with Egg

Heat a small frying pan and add oil, onion, apple and salt and pepper. Cook over medium heat until onions are translucent, add turkey and sprinkle with sage and parsley. Stir until well mixed and make a well in the center of pan and add egg. Cook until egg white is firm.	½ cup cooked turkey, cubed ¼ cup minced onion ¼ cup chopped apple Salt and pepper to taste ¼ teaspoon ground sage 1 teaspoon dried parsley 1 teaspoon canola oil 1 egg

Five Minute Frittata

Oil a microwave safe pie pan and add onion and green pepper. Cover and microwave on high for 1 minute. Beat eggs lightly and stir into onions and peppers. Season with salt and pepper and sprinkle with parsley. Cover and microwave for 1 to 2 minutes until a knife inserted in center comes out clean. Let stand for 3 minutes before cutting into serving pieces.	1 tablespoon extra virgin olive oil ½ cup chopped onion ¼ cup chopped green pepper ¼ cup chopped fresh parsley Salt and pepper to taste 4 eggs

Farm Fresh Omelet

Use half the oil to sauté the mushrooms with the lemon juice for one minute. Add the scallions and peppers and season with salt and pepper. When vegetables are done remove to a separate dish. Whisk eggs until light and frothy. Heat remaining oil in pan and add eggs. Cook over medium heat using a spatula to lift eggs as they set and allow uncooked eggs to move to the bottom of the pan. When eggs are almost done, spoon mushroom mixture on half of the eggs and fold over to form the omelet. Place on serving dish and sprinkle with parsley.

1 tablespoon extra virgin olive oil, divided

½ cup scallions, sliced

¼ cup red pepper, diced

2 tablespoons fresh parsley, minced

½ cup sliced fresh mushrooms

1 teaspoon lemon juice

3 eggs

Salt and pepper to taste

Egg White Omelet

If you are watching your cholesterol consumption, you can prepare the omelet using one whole egg and three egg whites whipped together. Follow the recipe above.

Creamy Spiced Oatmeal

Put the oats and lemon juice in a bowl and cover with water. Let soak overnight. Drain and rinse in a sieve with cold water. In a 1-quart microwave safe bowl, put oats, salt raisins and spices with 2 cups water. Microwave, uncovered, for six minutes at 50% power. Add almond milk and honey to serve.	1 cup steel cut oats 1 tablespoon lemon juice Pinch of salt ¼ cup dried cranberries ¼ teaspoon cinnamon ⅛ teaspoon powdered ginger ⅛ teaspoon ground cardamom 1 tablespoon honey ¼ cup almond milk 1 tablespoon sliced almonds

Hot Breakfast Rice

Combine all ingredients in a microwave safe bowl. Cover and microwave at half power for 1 minute or until heated through.	1 cup cooked brown rice ½ teaspoon cinnamon ¼ cup dried cherries or blueberries Pinch of salt ½ cup low-fat milk 1 teaspoon honey

Lunch Recipes

Shrimp Fried Rice

In a large frying pan sauté onion in canola oil, add garlic and red pepper and sauté for a minute. Add shrimp, peas, cabbage, pepper flakes and tamari and stir well.

Break rice into separate grains as you add to pan. Cook until peas are done and rice is warmed through. Garnish with scallions and serve.

1 cup cooked, peeled shrimp

¼ cup frozen peas

1 carrot, grated

1 small onion, sliced thin and quartered

1 clove garlic, crushed

¼ cup sweet red pepper, sliced thin

½ cup cabbage, sliced thin

3 tablespoons tamari sauce

1 tablespoon canola oil

¼ teaspoon red pepper flakes

1½ cups cooked and cooled brown rice

1 scallion sliced thin

Sizzling Stir Fry

Slice chicken into bite size and marinate for an hour in plastic bag with lemon juice, soy sauce, garlic, red pepper flakes and honey.

Heat wok or large frying pan, add oil, onions and mushrooms and stir constantly over high heat for one minute. Add chicken and all marinade and red pepper flakes. After one minute add frozen peas and oyster sauce and cook for 1 more minute or until snow peas are heated.

Garnish with scallions and parsley and serve over brown rice.

2 skinless, boneless chicken breasts

1 tablespoon fresh lemon juice

2 tablespoons soy sauce

2 cloves garlic, crushed

¼ teaspoon red pepper flakes

1 teaspoon honey

2 tablespoons canola oil

1 onion, sliced thin and quartered

1 red pepper, sliced in matchsticks

½ cup sliced fresh mushrooms

1 package frozen snow peas

1 tablespoon oyster sauce

2 scallions, sliced thin

2 tablespoons minced parsley

No Fail Brown Rice

In a microwave safe 4 quart casserole, microwave water and salt for 4 minutes on high.

Add rice and stir. Microwave on high for 5 minutes uncovered. Set microwave for 50% power and cook uncovered for 20 to 30 minutes. Check for doneness at 20 minutes. If pan is dry add water 2 tablespoons at a time. Check often until done.

Rice varies by age and variety so cooking time is approximate. When done, cover rice and fluff with fork before serving.

2 cups brown rice, rinsed and cleaned

3¾ cups water

½ teaspoon salt

Tropical Shrimp Salad

Place shrimp in a medium bowl and toss with lemon juice and zest. Stir in cilantro, avocado and salsa. Serve over chopped lettuce or roll shrimp salad into whole leaves.

1 cup cocktail shrimp, cooked and cooled

1 tablespoon fresh lemon juice

1 teaspoon lemon zest

2 tablespoons chopped cilantro

½ avocado, peeled and diced

¼ cup prepared fruit salsa

Romaine lettuce leaves

Chicken Salad Wrap

Mix first five ingredients and serve over chopped lettuce or roll salad into whole leaves.	1 cooked chicken breast, shredded
	2 tablespoons minced onion
	2 tablespoons minced celery
	2 tablespoons minced parsley
	2 tablespoons Balsamic vinaigrette
	Romaine lettuce leaves

Harvest Turkey Soup

In a large saucepan, sauté carrot, celery and onion in oil until onion becomes translucent. Add broth and sweet potato and bring to a boil then reduce heat and simmer until potato is tender. Add peas and turkey and heat thoroughly.	3 cups chicken broth
	½ cup frozen peas, thawed
	⅓ cup thinly sliced carrot
	⅓ cup sliced celery
Garnish with minced parsley.	2 tablespoons chopped onions
	½ cup diced fresh sweet potato
	½ cup diced cooked turkey
	2 teaspoons extra virgin olive oil
	1 tablespoon minced fresh parsley

Manhattan Clam Chowder

In a large saucepan, cook the onion, celery, green pepper and garlic in oil for 10 to 12 minutes, stirring often. Add all ingredients, except parsley, and cook until heated through. Ladle into serving bowls and top with a sprinkle of parsley.

1 large yellow onion, chopped

3 stalks celery, chopped

½ green pepper, seeded and chopped

1 large carrot, grated

1 clove garlic, crushed

2 tablespoons extra virgin olive oil

2 cups hot water

1 cup diced tomatoes, with juice

2 cups cooked and roughly chopped clams

½ teaspoon dried thyme

½ teaspoon dried basil

½ teaspoon fresh ground black pepper

2 teaspoons minced fresh parsley

Seafood Gumbo

In a large saucepan, sauté onion, celery, green pepper and garlic in olive oil until softened. Stir in V8, tomatoes, herbs and okra and bring to a boil.	1 onion, chopped
	2 stalks celery, sliced
	1 green pepper, chopped
	3 cloves garlic, crushed
Reduce heat, cover and simmer for 10 to 12 minutes. Add tilapia and cook for about 5 minutes then add shrimp. Stir well and when shrimp turns pink and opaque, remove from heat. Serve over rice.	1 tablespoon olive oil
	1 bottle spicy hot V8 juice
	1 cup diced tomatoes
	1 lb. fresh or frozen sliced okra
	1 lb. uncooked, peeled shrimp
	1 lb. tilapia filets, cut in cubes
	1 teaspoon dried Italian herbs
	3 cups cooked brown rice

Quick Turkey Chili

Sauté onion and garlic in oil until tender. Add turkey and salsa and mix well.	½ cup chopped onion
	1 clove garlic, crushed
	2 teaspoons olive oil
Simmer for 1 minute, add rice and heat through. Garnish with yogurt.	1 cup cooked turkey, diced
	1 cup cooked brown rice
	½ cup chunky salsa, mild, medium or hot according to preference
	2 tablespoons Greek yogurt

Gingered Catfish

In a small bowl, combine broth, soy sauce, ginger and cayenne. Cover and microwave at 50% power for 1 minute. Oil a casserole dish and arrange filets evenly. Sprinkle filets with scallions and drizzle evenly with sauce. Cover and microwave on high for 5 to 6 minutes until fish is opaque and flakes easily.

½ cup sliced scallions

1 tablespoon canola oil

¼ cup chicken broth

1 tablespoon soy sauce

1 teaspoon grated fresh ginger

¼ teaspoon cayenne pepper

4 6 oz. catfish filets

Oven Fish & Chips

Preheat oven to 400 degrees.

In a small baking tin, drizzle potatoes with canola oil and mix until evenly coated.

Sprinkle with Cajun seasoning to taste and bake for 10 minutes. Stir and bake for 10 more minutes or until outsides are browned, remove from oven, and cover with aluminum foil. Brush fish filets with milk, season with Cajun seasoning and roll in crushed cereal. Place on a nonstick baking pan and bake for 10 to 15 minutes.

1 sweet potato, peeled and cut into strips, ¾ inch

2 teaspoons canola oil

Cajun seasoned salt

¼ cup nonfat milk

½ cup whole grain breakfast cereal flakes, crushed

2 6 oz. catfish filets

Shrimp Salad in Tomato Cups

Lightly mix the shrimp and vegetables with the dressing and pile into tomato cups. Garnish with cilantro.	2 Large ripe tomatoes, cored and seeded 1 cup chopped cooked shrimp 2 tablespoons chopped cilantro 2 tablespoons chopped red sweet pepper 2 tablespoons chopped celery 3 tablespoons vinaigrette

Teriyaki Chicken with Roasted Veggies

Place all ingredients in a large zip lock bag and mix well. Marinate in refrigerator for an hour. Preheat oven to 400 degrees. In a large roasting pan, arrange chicken and vegetables in a single layer and drizzle with marinade. Bake for 20 minutes or until chicken is done.	1 lb. chicken breast tenders (fresh, unbreaded) 2 tablespoons canola oil 3 tablespoons teriyaki sauce 1 teaspoon fresh grated ginger 1 tablespoon fresh lemon juice ¼ teaspoon cayenne pepper ½ cup sliced mushrooms ½ cup sliced onions, quartered 1 red pepper, sliced in strips 1 small sweet potato, cubed

Spinach Salad with Citrus Vinaigrette

In salad bowl, toss spinach, separated onion rings, orange and carrot. In small bowl whisk together juice, vinegar, honey, mustard and olive oil. Serve garnished with egg wedges.

Leftover dressing can be stored in refrigerator.

2 cups fresh baby spinach, washed and dried

½ red onion, sliced in thin rings

1 seedless orange peeled and sliced in rounds

½ cup grated carrot

¼ cup orange juice

3 tablespoons red wine vinegar

2 teaspoons honey

1 tablespoon Dijon mustard

1 tablespoon olive oil

2 hardboiled eggs, peeled and cut in wedges

Quick Rotisserie Chicken Soup

Cut chicken in half lengthwise so that it will easily be covered by stock. Place in a large, heavy stockpot. Add the rest of the ingredients, except for the parsley. Bring to a boil, lower heat to a simmer, cover and cook for forty-five minutes. Remove chicken, pull all meat from bones, discarding the skin. Shred or chop chicken, return to pot to reheat and serve with a sprinkling of fresh parsley.

1 fully cooked and seasoned rotisserie chicken

1 cup peeled baby carrots

½ cup chopped celery

1 cup fresh spinach leaves

4 cups chicken stock

2 tablespoons chopped fresh parsley

Dinner Recipes

Cod with Roasted Asparagus

Preheat oven to 400 degrees.

In shallow roasting pan, toss asparagus with oil and sprinkle with salt. Arrange in a single layer and place in preheated oven.

Oil another shallow pan and arrange fish. In small bowl mix lemon juice and teriyaki and drizzle evenly over fish. Bake for approximately 12 minutes or until thickest part of fish is opaque and flakes easily. Garnish with lemon.

1 bunch fresh asparagus, washed, trimmed and dried

2 teaspoons olive oil

¼ teaspoon sea salt

2 6 oz. cod filets, fresh or thawed

1 teaspoon olive oil

1 teaspoon lemon juice

1 tablespoon teriyaki sauce

Lemon slices for garnish

Scampi with Green Rice

In 2 quart microwave casserole, heat vegetable broth and water for 4 minutes on high.

Stir in brown rice and microwave uncovered on high for five minutes. Cook uncovered at 50% power for 20 to 30 minutes until rice is tender and liquid is absorbed. Add a couple tablespoons water if rice is dry and has not finished cooking. Cover and keep warm.

Cook broccoli in microwave until tender and drain. Mix rice, broccoli and parsley together. Heat a large frying pan to medium high, add oil, shrimp, garlic and red pepper flakes. Sauté over medium heat until shrimp turns pink, tossing to cook evenly.

Stir in lemon juice and zest and serve over rice.

1 cup long grain brown rice

2 cups vegetable broth

½ cup water

1 10 oz. package frozen, chopped broccoli

½ cup minced fresh parsley

1 tablespoon lemon juice

Zest from 1 lemon

1 lb. large shrimp, tails left on and dried on paper towel

1 tablespoon olive oil

2 cloves garlic, crushed

½ teaspoon red pepper flakes

Roast Chicken

Preheat oven to 350 degrees.

Wash chicken with cold water inside and out. Drain and place on rack in roaster pan.

Put onion, garlic, lemon and sage inside the cavity and roast for 25 minutes per pound. Meat thermometer inserted in thickest part of thigh should register 180 degrees.

Allow to rest for 10 minutes before carving for serving. Let chicken cool until easily handled. Discard skin and cut meat into serving portions and store in freezer in zip lock bags. This is an economical way to have cooked chicken on hand for use in many recipes.

1 3 to 4 lb. broiler fryer chicken

1 onion, cut in eighths

4 cloves garlic, sliced

½ lemon

1 teaspoon rubbed sage

Turkey Patties

In a bowl combine the egg, crumbs, celery, onion and seasonings. Mix well. Crumble the turkey into the bowl and mix well to combine. Form into 4 inch patties, 1 inch thick. Brush both sides with Worcestershire sauce. Heat frying pan over medium heat, add oil and cook patties for five minutes on each side.

1 lb. lean ground turkey breast

1 egg, lightly beaten

½ cup whole grain cereal, crushed finely

⅓ cup finely chopped celery

⅓ cup finely chopped onion

2 teaspoons dried parsley

1 teaspoon dried oregano

½ teaspoon salt

¼ teaspoon pepper

2 teaspoons Worcestershire sauce

1 tablespoon olive oil

Turkey Fajitas

Slice turkey into strips. Heat oil in frying pan and add half the onion, the green and red pepper and jalapeno. Sauté for five minutes and add turkey. Brown meat on all sides and add salsa. Simmer for twenty minutes or until done.

Wrap tortillas in damp paper towels and microwave for 15 to 30 seconds. Spoon turkey and vegetables onto tortilla, add remaining raw onion, chopped lettuce, Greek yogurt and additional salsa as desired.

½ lb. fresh turkey breast

½ sweet red pepper, sliced

½ green pepper, diced

1 onion, sliced and divided

1 Jalapeño pepper, seeded and chopped

20 green olives sliced

1 tablespoon olive oil

2 tablespoons prepared salsa

2 whole grain tortillas

Additional salsa and Greek Yogurt

Chopped lettuce

Rosemary Chicken

Place all ingredients in a zip lock bag and marinate in refrigerator for one hour.

Preheat oven to 350 degrees. Place chicken in a single layer in a baking pan and bake for 40 to 50 minutes, spooning marinade over meat every 15 minutes.

1 pound chicken breast filets

1 tablespoon dried rosemary, crushed

4 cloves garlic, sliced

1 tablespoon lemon juice

1 tablespoon olive oil

1 teaspoon balsamic vinegar

Salt and pepper

Roast Turkey Breast

Preheat oven to 350 degrees.

Place turkey on rack in roasting pan. Pull skin away from breast leaving bottom edge intact.

Mix marinade in small bowl and rub between skin and meat. Bake uncovered for 2½ to 3 hours, basting occasionally, until meat thermometer registers 170 degrees. Let rest, covered, for at least 10 minutes before carving. Remove and discard skin. Carve into serving portions and freeze in freezer bags for use in recipes that call for cooked turkey.

1 bone-in turkey breast (about 8 lbs)

1 teaspoon salt

2 cloves garlic, crushed

1 teaspoon dried thyme

1 teaspoon rubbed sage

1 teaspoon pepper

3 tablespoons olive oil

2 tablespoons lemon juice

Chicken Cacciatore

Season chicken with salt and pepper. Heat oil in a large pot over medium-high heat. Add chicken and sauté about 5 minutes on each side until browned. Remove chicken to a plate and set aside. Add bell pepper, onion and garlic and sauté over medium heat for 5 minutes or until reduced. Add tomatoes with their juice, broth, capers and oregano. Return the chicken to the pan and turn to coat them in sauce. Simmer over medium low heat until the chicken is cooked through, about 20 minutes. Serve over brown rice and garnish with basil.

4 boneless, skinless chicken breasts

¼ teaspoon salt

½ teaspoon freshly ground black pepper

2 tablespoons olive oil

1 large red bell pepper, chopped

1 onion, chopped

3 garlic cloves, finely chopped

¾ cup dry white wine

2 cups chopped fresh tomatoes with juice

¾ cup reduced-sodium chicken broth

3 tablespoons drained capers

1 teaspoon dried oregano leaves

¼ cup coarsely chopped fresh basil leaves

Seared Salmon with Greens

Season the fish on both sides with salt and pepper. In a sauté pan heat 2 tablespoons of oil and place the salmon, skin-side down, and cook without moving until the skin is crispy (about 4 to 5 minutes). Reduce heat. Turn salmon over and cook for another 3 to 4 minutes.

In another pan, heat one tablespoon oil over medium heat. Add garlic and shallots and sauté for 4 minutes. Add the beans, stock and spinach and cook for 3 minutes, tossing to wilt all the spinach and heat the beans through.

- 2 6-ounce salmon filets, with skin
- Salt and pepper
- 3 tablespoon olive oil
- 1 teaspoon minced garlic
- 2 teaspoons diced shallot
- 1 bag fresh baby spinach
- 1 cup fish stock
- 8 ounces canned cannellini beans, drained

Savory Chicken and Mushrooms

Preheat oven to 400 degrees.

In a large skillet, brown chicken on both sides in oil. Place chicken in a shallow baking dish.

Add mushrooms to skillet and sauté for 5 minutes. Deglaze pan with broth and add salt, pepper and thyme. Pour over chicken. Cover and bake for 20 to 25 minutes or until a meat thermometer registers 170 degrees.

- 2 cups sliced fresh mushrooms
- 3 tablespoons extra virgin olive oil
- 6 boneless chicken breasts
- 1/4 teaspoon salt
- 1/4 teaspoon pepper
- 1 teaspoon dried thyme
- 1 cup chicken broth

Oriental Chicken Salad

Combine first six ingredients in salad bowl, whisking well. Add greens, chicken, carrots and snow peas and toss gently to coat the greens. Sprinkle with almonds and serve.

1 tablespoon low-sodium soy sauce

1 tablespoon rice vinegar

1 tablespoon lemon juice

1 tablespoon canola oil

1 teaspoon grated fresh ginger

1 teaspoon honey

1 bag gourmet salad greens

2 cups chopped cooked chicken

1 cup matchstick-cut carrots

1 cup snow peas, ends trimmed

¼ cup sliced almonds

Shrimp Salad with Capers

Add all ingredients except lettuce to a medium bowl and mix well. Serve over lettuce.

1 pound cooked small shrimp, peeled and deveined

2 teaspoons capers, rinsed and chopped

1 tablespoon minced onion

2 teaspoons fresh lemon juice

1 teaspoon olive oil

¼ teaspoon chopped fresh dill

Salt and pepper to taste

Romaine lettuce leaves

Cheesy Spinach Salad

In serving bowl, layer half the spinach and half the cottage cheese and walnuts; repeat. In small bowl, whisk the remaining ingredients and drizzle over spinach. Toss to coat evenly.

- 2 cups fresh baby spinach leaves
- ½ cup nonfat cottage cheese
- ½ cup chopped walnuts
- 2 tablespoons honey
- 2 tablespoons vinegar
- 1 teaspoon prepared horseradish
- ½ teaspoon Dijon mustard
- Salt and pepper to taste

Szechwan Chicken and Broccoli

Cut and separate broccoli florets from stems. Trim and peel stems and cut in small circles.

Bring a large pot of water to boil and add salt. Blanch broccoli for 1 minute then drain into colander and plunge into cold water bath to stop cooking. Drain and set aside. Mix vinegars, tamari, and honey and set aside. Heat a wok over high heat and add the canola oil, red pepper flakes, ginger , and scallions. Stir quickly for 30 seconds then add the sauce and simmer for another 30 seconds then add broccoli and chicken. Heat through and serve over rice.

- 1 bunch fresh broccoli
- ½ teaspoon salt
- 2 tablespoons rice vinegar
- 2 tablespoons tamari
- 1 tablespoon red wine vinegar
- 1 teaspoon honey
- 1 tablespoon canola oil
- ¼ teaspoon red pepper flakes
- 3 cloves garlic, minced
- 1 tablespoon fresh ginger, grated
- 2 cups cooked chicken, shredded
- 2 scallions, minced

Stuffed Acorn Squash

Preheat oven to 350 degrees. Poke inside of squash with a fork all over. Brush with olive oil and season with salt and pepper. Place on baking sheet and bake for 35 to 45 minutes until tender.

Meanwhile prepare turkey hash, but omit the egg. When squash is cooked, stuff with hash and serve.

1 acorn squash, halved

1 teaspoon olive oil

Salt and pepper

1 recipe Turkey Hash (see Lunch recipes) without egg

Dessert Recipes

Blueberry Crisp

Preheat oven to 350 degrees.
Lightly oil and 9-inch glass pie
plate with canola oil.

In a large bowl combine kudzu,
blueberries, cinnamon, ginger,
lemon juice and honey and set
aside. Pulse Crunchy Granola in
food processor for a few seconds to
make a crumbly crust.

Pour blueberries into prepared pie
plate and top evenly with granola.
Push down into fruit with a large
spoon. Bake for 25 minutes.
Cool for about 15 minutes before
serving.

1 teaspoon kudzu powder
dissolved in 2 tablespoons
cold water

2 10 oz. bags frozen organic
blueberries

1 teaspoon cinnamon

1 teaspoon fresh ginger,
grated

Pinch sea salt

1 tablespoon fresh lemon
juice

2 tablespoons honey

3 cups Crunchy Granola (see
Breakfast Recipes)

Thumbprint Cookies

Preheat oven to 350 degrees. Line cookie pan with parchment paper.

Use a food processor with metal blade to grind almonds into coarse flour, about 2 minutes. Add oats, flour, cinnamon, ginger, nutmeg and salt and process for one more minute. Add oil, honey and vanilla extract and continue to process until dough forms a ball. Wrap dough in plastic wrap set aside for 15 minutes at room temperature.

Using a tablespoon of dough, form balls and place on cookie sheet. Make a thumb print in each cookie and fill with Overnight Jam. Bake about 15 minutes until cookie bottoms are browned.

1 cup raw almonds

1 cup rolled oats

1 cup organic spelt flour

½ teaspoon cinnamon

½ teaspoon powdered ginger

⅛ teaspoon nutmeg

¼ teaspoon salt

½ cup canola oil

½ cup honey

1 teaspoon vanilla extract

Overnight Jam (see below) for filling

Overnight Jam

Tightly pack the dried fruits into the measuring cups. Roughly chop all fruits and put in bowl with salt and cover with water. Cover bowl and refrigerate for 12 hours or overnight until fruit is plump. Drain excess water and place is food processor or blender. Blend until you have a thick, chunky jam, Store tightly sealed in refrigerator for up to 2 weeks.

¼ cup dried apricots

¼ cup dried cherries

½ cup dried apples

Pinch of salt

Parfait with Ginger Cream

Put water, almonds, honey, lemon juice, salt, extracts, ginger and cinnamon and peaches into blender. Blend until very smooth and creamy. Alternate layers of cream and fresh fruit in parfait glasses and garnish top with cream and a berry or fruit slice. Chill and serve.

2 cups fresh fruit in season, washed and sliced as needed

1 cup raw blanched almonds

2 tablespoons honey

1 teaspoon fresh lemon juice

¼ teaspoon salt

¼ teaspoon almond extract

½ teaspoon vanilla extract

1 teaspoon grated fresh ginger

¼ teaspoon cinnamon

2 ripe peaches, peeled and sliced

1 cup water

Rice Pudding

Combine rice, milk, raisins and honey in saucepan and simmer for 20 minutes stirring frequently. Remove from heat and add cinnamon and vanilla and lemon zest and stir well. Toast coconut in a dry skillet over low heat just until edges get golden. Spoon pudding into serving dish and sprinkle with toasted coconut. Serve warm or cold.

3 cups cooked brown rice

2 cups coconut milk

1 cup almond milk

½ cup honey

1 teaspoon vanilla extract

Zest of 1 lemon, grated

1 teaspoon cinnamon

Fruity Greek Spread

Add all ingredients except olive oil to a blender and pulse for one minute. With the blender running, slowly add the olive oil and process until smooth and creamy. Place in serving container on platter with fruits and veggies.

2 cups orange or peach Greek yogurt

1 tablespoon white miso

¼ cup fresh lemon juice

3 tablespoons fresh orange juice

2 teaspoons salt

½ cup honey

1 teaspoon fresh grated nutmeg

½ teaspoon cinnamon

1 tablespoon powdered ginger

1 tablespoon orange zest

1 tablespoon lemon zest

¼ cup extra virgin olive oil

An assortment of firm fresh fruits and veggies

Frozen Fruit Cream with Chocolate Chips

Put all ingredients in a blender and blend on medium for about 30 seconds. Then blend on high for another 30 seconds until it is as thick as ice cream. Serve immediately.

3 frozen bananas cut into 1 inch chunks

1 cup almond milk

½ cup raw walnuts

3 tablespoons raw cacao nibs

1 tablespoon honey

1 teaspoon vanilla extract

Pinch of salt

Frozen Banana Treats

Grind the almonds into a fine meal and put into a small bowl. Mix the carob, agave and cinnamon in another bowl until it is completely blended. Slice the bananas into 1 inch pieces. Roll each piece in the carob until coated and then roll in the almond meal. Place on a cookie sheet in a single layer, not touching, and freeze for 4 hours. Store in ziplock bags in the freezer for no more than two weeks.

½ cup raw almonds

¼ cup carob powder

¼ cup agave nectar

½ teaspoon cinnamon

3 bananas

Mango Almond Parfait

Crush the granola and walnuts in a Ziploc bag with a rolling pin to make coarse crumbs. In two parfait glasses, layer 2 tablespoons granola and a layer of mango. 20 minutes before serving, fill each glass with ½ cup yogurt and a dusting of cinnamon.

1 ripe mango, peeled, pitted and diced

½ cup Crunchy Granola (see Breakfast recipes)

¼ cup walnuts

Pinch of cinnamon

1 cup vanilla Greek yogurt

Lemon Drops

Put all ingredients in a food processer and blend for 15 seconds. Scrape down and blend again for another 15 seconds. Repeat again and a dough ball should form. Roll dough into 1-inch balls and store tightly sealed in refrigerator for a week or freeze for up to a month.

4 teaspoons lemon zest

2 tablespoons lemon juice

1 cup raw walnuts

½ cup raw sesame seeds

Dash of salt

Spiced Halvah

Process sesame seeds for 1½ minutes in food processor to produce a slightly coarse meal. Pour into a large bowl and add the spices and salt and mix well. Slowly add the honey, sesame butter and vanilla and knead until well mixed and a stiff dough forms. Line a 9 × 9 inch pan with plastic wrap and press the dough evenly into the pan.

Cover and refrigerate to let dough stiffen, then cut into 1 inch squares. Store in ziplock bag in refrigerator for up to 3 weeks.

1 cup raw sesame seeds

½ teaspoon cinnamon

¼ teaspoon cardamom

Dash of salt

½ cup honey

2 tablespoons sesame butter

1 teaspoon vanilla extract

Fudgy Walnut Brownies

Soak the dates in water to cover for 3 hours. Blend the walnuts to a coarse meal in a food processor.

Drain the dates and add them and the oats, almond butter, cocoa, cinnamon and salt. Blend to form a moist dough, about 30 seconds. Lightly oil an 8-inch square pan and press the dough into the pan.

Cover and freeze for 2 hours. Remove and cut the brownies into small squares and store tightly sealed in refrigerator for up to 2 weeks.

1½ cups raw walnuts

8 pitted dates

1 cup rolled oats

½ cup almond butter

½ cup carob powder

¼ teaspoon cinnamon

Dash of salt

Canola oil

Frozen Fudge

Soak the dates in water and cover for 4 hours. Drain dates and put all ingredients in food processor.

Process for 30 seconds until a moist dough forms. Oil an 8-inch square pan and press the dough evenly into the pan. Cover and freeze for 4 hours to harden. Cut into 1½ inch squares and store tightly sealed in freezer for up to 3 months.

12 pitted dates

1 cup almond butter

1 cup carob powder

2 tablespoons honey

½ teaspoon vanilla extract

Dash of salt

No-Bake Vanilla Nut Cookies

Blend all ingredients in food processor for about a minute. Transfer to a bowl. Mixture will be oily. Pinch off pieces and roll into 2 inch balls. Press slightly to flatten into cookies. Store tightly sealed for 3 weeks in refrigerator.	2 cups raw walnuts 1 cup uncooked oats ¼ cup honey 1 teaspoon vanilla extract ¼ teaspoon nutmeg

Mexicali Fudge

Put all ingredients in a large bowl and stir until a stiff, lumpy ball forms. Coat the bottom of an 8 inch square pan with oil and spread in the fudge. Cover and freeze for an hour. Remove from freezer and let it soften for 15 to 20 minutes. Cut into 1½ inch squares and store in refrigerator for up to 2 months.	½ cup canola oil ½ cup dried blueberries ½ cup dried cherries, chopped 1 cup cocoa powder ½ cup almond butter 2 tablespoons agave nectar ½ teaspoon chili powder 1 teaspoon cinnamon ½ teaspoon cayenne pepper Dash salt Canola oil

Snacks

Almond Milk

Soak nuts overnight in water to cover. Drain and rinse and place in blender with water and honey.	1½ cups raw almonds
	4 cups water
	1 tablespoon honey
Blend on high for two minutes. Strain the milk using a nut milk bag. Store in refrigerator for 2 to 3 days. Shake to mix before serving.	

Virgin Mojito

Blend all ingredients except garnish in blender for 30 seconds. Garnish and serve immediately.	4 cups cold seedless watermelon chunks
	Juice of 1 lime
	1 tablespoon honey
	8 fresh mint leaves
	4 ice cubes
	Mint sprigs for garnish

Strawberry Ice Cream

Put all ingredients into a blender and blend on medium for 30 seconds. Clear blades if necessary and blend another 30 seconds. Serve immediately.	1 cup almond milk 5 dried apricots 2 cups frozen strawberries 2 frozen bananas cut in 1 inch chunks 1 tablespoon honey 1 teaspoon vanilla extract Dash of salt

Cantaloupe Slushy

Remove cantaloupe from freezer a half-hour before preparing slushy. Place all ingredients in blender and blend on high for 30 seconds. Serve immediately.	1 cantaloupe, peeled, cut into chunks and frozen ½ cup fresh orange juice 1 tablespoon honey 4 ice cubes

Bugs on a Log

Trim ends off celery and cut into serving pieces. Fill with cheese spread and press blueberries into the cheese.	2 stalks celery ¼ cup Fruity Cheese Spread (see Dessert Recipes) ¼ cup dried blueberries

Nutty Bugs on Logs

Trim ends off celery and cut into serving pieces. Fill with almond or sesame butter and press raisins into the filling.	2 stalks celery ¼ cup almond or sesame butter ¼ cup raisins

Apple Snack

Wash, core and slice apple and spread with nut butter for a healthy snack.	1 apple ½ cup almond or sesame nut butter

Spinach Dip

Cook spinach in microwave just until defrosted. Set aside to cool. Slice avocado in half and remove pit. Scoop flesh into food processor and sprinkle with lemon juice. Squeeze spinach until almost dry and add to processor with onion and salt. Process for 1 minute until smooth. Keeps for up to two days in refrigerator. Try other fresh veggies like cucumber, radish and zucchini for dipping.	1 ripe Hass avocado 1 small onion, chopped 1 tablespoon fresh lemon juice 1 10 oz. package frozen chopped spinach 1 teaspoon salt Fresh celery and carrot sticks for dipping

Curry Onion Dip

Put all ingredients in a food processor and blend until smooth, scraping down sides as needed. Will keep in refrigerator for up to a week.

1 cup raw almonds

1 onion, chopped

3 tablespoons fresh lime juice

3 tablespoons extra virgin olive oil

1 teaspoon curry powder

½ teaspoon salt

½ teaspoon pepper

½ teaspoon paprika

Fresh vegetable crudities for dipping

Veggie Dip

Put all ingredients in food processor and blend for 1 minute until thick and smooth. Store tightly sealed in refrigerator for no more than 5 days.

¼ cup fresh parsley leaves, chopped

1 red sweet pepper, chopped

½ cup chopped onion

¼ cup extra virgin olive oil

1 tablespoon fresh lemon juice

1 tablespoon tamari sauce

½ teaspoon black pepper

Dash salt

¼ teaspoon cayenne pepper

Fresh veggies for dipping

Red Pepper Hummus

Place all ingredients in food processor and process until smooth. Will keep in refrigerator for four days.	1 can chickpeas, rinsed and drained
	2 cloves garlic, crushed
	2 tablespoons lemon juice
	¼ cup sesame butter or tahini
	½ cup roasted red sweet pepper, chopped
	Pinch of salt
	1 teaspoon paprika
	2 tablespoons extra virgin olive oil
	Vegetable crudités for dipping

Deviled Eggs

Remove yolks from eggs and mix with hummus or onion dip in small bowl. Spoon yolk mixture back into egg whites and dust with paprika.	2 hardboiled eggs, peeled and halved
	2 tablespoons Red Pepper Hummus or Curry Onion Dip (see recipes)
	Paprika

Sweet Potato Chips

Preheat oven to 375 degrees. In a bowl, combine the potato and oil, tossing to coat evenly. Spread the chips in a single layer on a greased baking sheet and sprinkle evenly with seasoned salt. Bake for 10 to 12 minutes or until edges of potato start to brown.	1 sweet potato, peeled and cut into ¼ inch rounds 2 teaspoons olive oil ½ teaspoon Cajun seasoned salt

Savory Mixed Nuts

Preheat oven to 350 degrees. Place nuts in a bowl and drizzle with oil. Toss until evenly coated then sprinkle with seasoned salt and toss again. Place in a single layer on a large baking sheet and bake for 20 minutes. Stir after ten minutes.	2 cups raw nuts like almonds, walnuts or pecans 1 tablespoon light olive oil 1 teaspoon seasoned salt (choose your favorite flavor)

Shrimp Cocktail

Mix horseradish, tomato paste, and agave nectar vigorously. Squeeze juice into sauce in a small dish. Serve chilled with shrimp.	6 cooked shrimp, peeled and chilled 2 tablespoons horseradish 1 teaspoon tomato paste ½ teaspoon agave nectar 1 teaspoon fresh lemon juice

The
Belly Fat Diet
Shopping Guide

The Belly Fat Diet Shopping Guide

Vegetables

- ☐ Alfalfa sprouts
- ☐ Arugula
- ☐ Bamboo shoots
- ☐ Bean sprouts
- ☐ Beet greens
- ☐ Beets
- ☐ Bell peppers
- ☐ Bok choy
- ☐ Broccoli
- ☐ Broccoflower
- ☐ Brussels sprouts
- ☐ Cabbage
- ☐ Carrots
- ☐ Cauliflower
- ☐ Chard (Swiss & red)

- ☐ Chinese cabbage
- ☐ Chives
- ☐ Collard greens
- ☐ Garlic
- ☐ Green onions
- ☐ Green peas
- ☐ Greens
- ☐ Horseradish
- ☐ Kale
- ☐ Leeks
- ☐ Lettuce (preferably dark, leafy varieties)
- ☐ Lima beans
- ☐ Mushrooms
- ☐ Mustard greens
- ☐ Onions
- ☐ Parsley
- ☐ Peppers, preferably orange or red
- ☐ Pumpkin
- ☐ Sauerkraut
- ☐ Shallot
- ☐ Snow peas
- ☐ Soy beans
- ☐ Spinach
- ☐ Summer squash
- ☐ Sweet potato & yam
- ☐ Tomato
- ☐ Turnip greens
- ☐ Watercress
- ☐ Water chestnuts
- ☐ Winter squash

Fruits

- ☐ Acai berry — also called the Acai fruit
- ☐ Apples
- ☐ Apricot
- ☐ Avocado
- ☐ Banana
- ☐ Blackberries
- ☐ Black raspberries
- ☐ Blueberries
- ☐ Boysenberries
- ☐ Cantaloupe
- ☐ Cherries
- ☐ Clementines
- ☐ Coconut
- ☐ Dates
- ☐ Figs
- ☐ Grapefruit
- ☐ Grapes
- ☐ Guava
- ☐ Honeydew melon
- ☐ Honey pomelo
- ☐ Jujube — a subtropical fruit
- ☐ Lemon
- ☐ Lime
- ☐ Lingonberries
- ☐ Mango
- ☐ Nectarines
- ☐ Oranges
- ☐ Papaya
- ☐ Peaches
- ☐ Pears

- ☐ Persimmon
- ☐ Pineapple
- ☐ Pitaya or Dragon fruit
- ☐ Plums
- ☐ Pomegranate
- ☐ Raspberries
- ☐ Star fruit
- ☐ Strawberries
- ☐ Tangerines
- ☐ Ugli fruit
- ☐ Watermelon

Fish and Seafood

Oily Fish Varieties

- ☐ Salmon
- ☐ Trout
- ☐ Mackerel
- ☐ Herring, fresh
- ☐ Sardines, in water or olive oil
- ☐ Pilchards
- ☐ Kipper
- ☐ Eel
- ☐ Whitebait
- ☐ Tuna (fresh is best but packed in water is okay, too)
- ☐ Anchovies
- ☐ Swordfish
- ☐ Bloater
- ☐ Cacha

- ☐ Carp
- ☐ Hilsa
- ☐ Jack fish
- ☐ Katla
- ☐ Orange roughy
- ☐ Pangas
- ☐ Sprats

Other Great Fish

- ☐ Cod
- ☐ Haddock
- ☐ Sole
- ☐ Flounder
- ☐ Snapper
- ☐ Catfish
- ☐ Skate
- ☐ Whiting
- ☐ Smelt

Shellfish, Mollusks and Misc.

- ☐ Shrimp
- ☐ Crab
- ☐ Lobster
- ☐ Crawfish
- ☐ Clams
- ☐ Oysters
- ☐ Scallops
- ☐ Prawns
- ☐ Octopus
- ☐ Squid

Meats and Poultry

- ☐ Lean beef steaks and roasts, trimmed of all visible fat (limit of one serving per week)
- ☐ Chicken breast, skin removed
- ☐ Ground chicken breast meat
- ☐ Turkey breast, skin removed
- ☐ Ground turkey breast meat
- ☐ Eggs

Dairy Products

- ☐ Skim, 1% or 2% milk
- ☐ Almond milk
- ☐ Low-fat or nonfat cottage cheese
- ☐ Low-fat or part-skim Mozzarella
- ☐ Greek Yogurt, probiotic if available

Grains

- ☐ Brown rice
- ☐ Whole grain oats
- ☐ Whole grain hot and cold cereals, no sugar added
- ☐ Barley
- ☐ Quinoa
- ☐ Whole grain bread
- ☐ Whole grain, whole wheat flour
- ☐ Whole grain wrap or tortilla

Nuts, Seeds and Oils

- ☐ Canola oil
- ☐ Olive oil
- ☐ Almonds
- ☐ Brazil nuts
- ☐ Pecans
- ☐ Pine nuts
- ☐ Poppy seeds
- ☐ Pumpkin seeds
- ☐ Sesame seeds
- ☐ Walnuts
- ☐ Almond butter
- ☐ Sesame butter

Other Allowed Foods

- ☐ Balsamic vinegar
- ☐ Rice vinegar
- ☐ Mustard
- ☐ Horseradish
- ☐ Hot sauce
- ☐ Soy sauce
- ☐ Teriyaki sauce
- ☐ Herbs and Curry
- ☐ Nori (Seaweed paper)
- ☐ Whey or Soy protein powder, no sugar
- ☐ Flax seed

- ☐ Psyllium husk
- ☐ Bran flakes
- ☐ Brown or white sugar
- ☐ Honey
- ☐ Agave nectar
- ☐ Dried blueberries
- ☐ Dried cranberries
- ☐ Dried cherries
- ☐ Dried apricots
- ☐ Dried peaches
- ☐ Dried pineapple
- ☐ Dried figs
- ☐ Green tea
- ☐ Black tea
- ☐ Coffee
- ☐ Water (lots!)

Sweet Treats

- ☐ Frozen fruit pops, no sugar
- ☐ Sorbet, no sugar
- ☐ Dark chocolate, min. 66% cacao
- ☐ Nonfat pudding

The Shopping Guide

You can use this guide to help plan your grocery shopping or take it with you to use as a section-by-section guide.

For the most part, shopping for the Belly Fat Diet is pretty straightforward: shop around the edges of the store, where the produce, meat, seafood and dairy sections are usually situated. There isn't a whole lot for you in the middle, where the grocery items, convenience foods and snacks are located. We'll cover those areas, too, but you'll be shopping mostly from the perimeter of the store.

The Produce Section

This is one of only two departments where you have almost free reign; the other is the seafood counter. However, there are some things to keep in mind when choosing your produce.

Buy organic as much as you can afford to. If you're on a tight budget, buy organic fruits and veggies if you'll be eating them raw with peel intact, but you can buy traditional varieties if you'll be peeling or cooking them before you eat.

Try to get a wide variety of the power produce items. These are greens that are dark and leafy and fruits, berries and veggies that are dark red, orange or yellow. They have the highest antioxidant and phytonutrient content.

Remember, no white potatoes or corn.

The Seafood Section

When buying fish, opt for the oily varieties first to get that rich Omega-3 content.

When choosing any fish, shellfish and mollusks, fresh is best, even if you'll be freezing it. Make sure it hasn't been thawed from frozen. If it has, you'll need to eat it right away or cook it before you can safely freeze it again.

Fish from the frozen food section is okay to buy, as long as it contains no breading, coatings or sauces.

The Meat Section

Here again, buy organic, grass-fed meats and poultry if at all possible. You'll avoid the hormones, additives and other things your body doesn't need. Kosher products are also a good way to go.

You can buy chicken and turkey breasts with the skin and ribs removed or save a good deal of money by removing them yourself. It isn't hard and only takes a few minutes. You can even use the skins and ribs for making your own stock.

When buying ground chicken or turkey, be sure the label says ground breast meat, not just ground chicken or turkey. Regular ground chicken and turkey often includes dark meat and skin and contain the same amount of fat as a juicy steak.

On the subject of beef, you're looking for leaner cuts of steak and roasts. Rounds and loins are some of the leaner cuts to consider.

The Dairy Section

Shopping here is pretty simple, since your choices are fairly limited to milk, almond milk, eggs (free range, organic and vegetarian), Greek yogurt (probiotic if available), mozzarella and cottage cheese, both in low or nonfat varieties. You can also find your nonfat pudding here, any flavor you like.

The Frozen Food Section

We've already mentioned that frozen seafood is okay to purchase.

You may also want to pick up frozen veggies without butter or sauce added and frozen fruits without syrup or added sugar.

Other foods you'll find here are frozen fruit bars (the kind with whole fruit, water and nothing else) and sorbet with no added sugar.

The Grocery or Middle Sections

There isn't much here for you, but you'll be picking up a few things. The less time you spend in the center of the store, the less time you'll have to be tempted by cookies, chips and other nasty tidbits. Those are for cheat days and you shouldn't buy them until cheat day. Having them in the house all week is a bad idea.

When buying sandwich bread, wraps or tortillas, make sure they're whole-grain. Whole wheat does not mean whole-grain, so read the labels carefully. Also, you want at least 6 grams of fiber in a slice of bread or it just isn't worth it. Make sure to check for high fructose corn syrup in the ingredients and put the bread back if it's there.

You'll want to pick up brown rice, quinoa, whole grain, steel cut oats and whole, multigrain hot and cold cereals in those aisles.

You can also pick up dried figs, dates, cherries, berries and other fruits here. Choose those without added sugar.

Other than the allowed condiments, oils, sugar, honey, tea, coffee, spices and herbs, there isn't much else for you here.